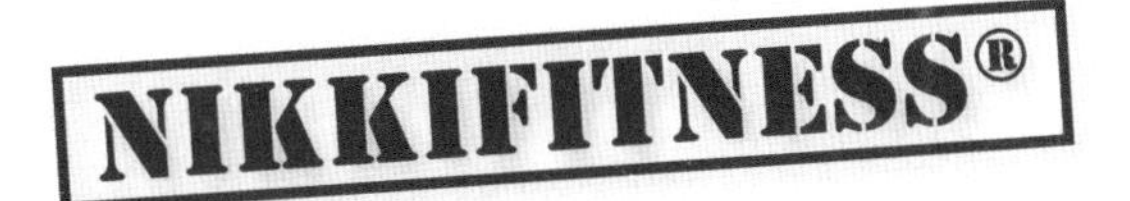

The Slimnastics® Workout

The Intense, No-Equipment Routine Combining Gymnastics, Plyometrics, and Advanced Yoga

PUBLISHED BY GT MEDIA

by Nicole Glor of NikkiFitness®

By Nicole Glor or NikkiFitness®: DVD Instructor, Former College Cheerleader, NYC Personal Trainer, Boot Camp Class Instructor, Yoga Teacher, Media Fitness Expert!

Published 2012 GT Media
Yoga Studio Photos by Adam Watstein,
Sharpshooter Pictures

ISBN: 1466497300
ISBN 13: 9781466497306

Table of Contents

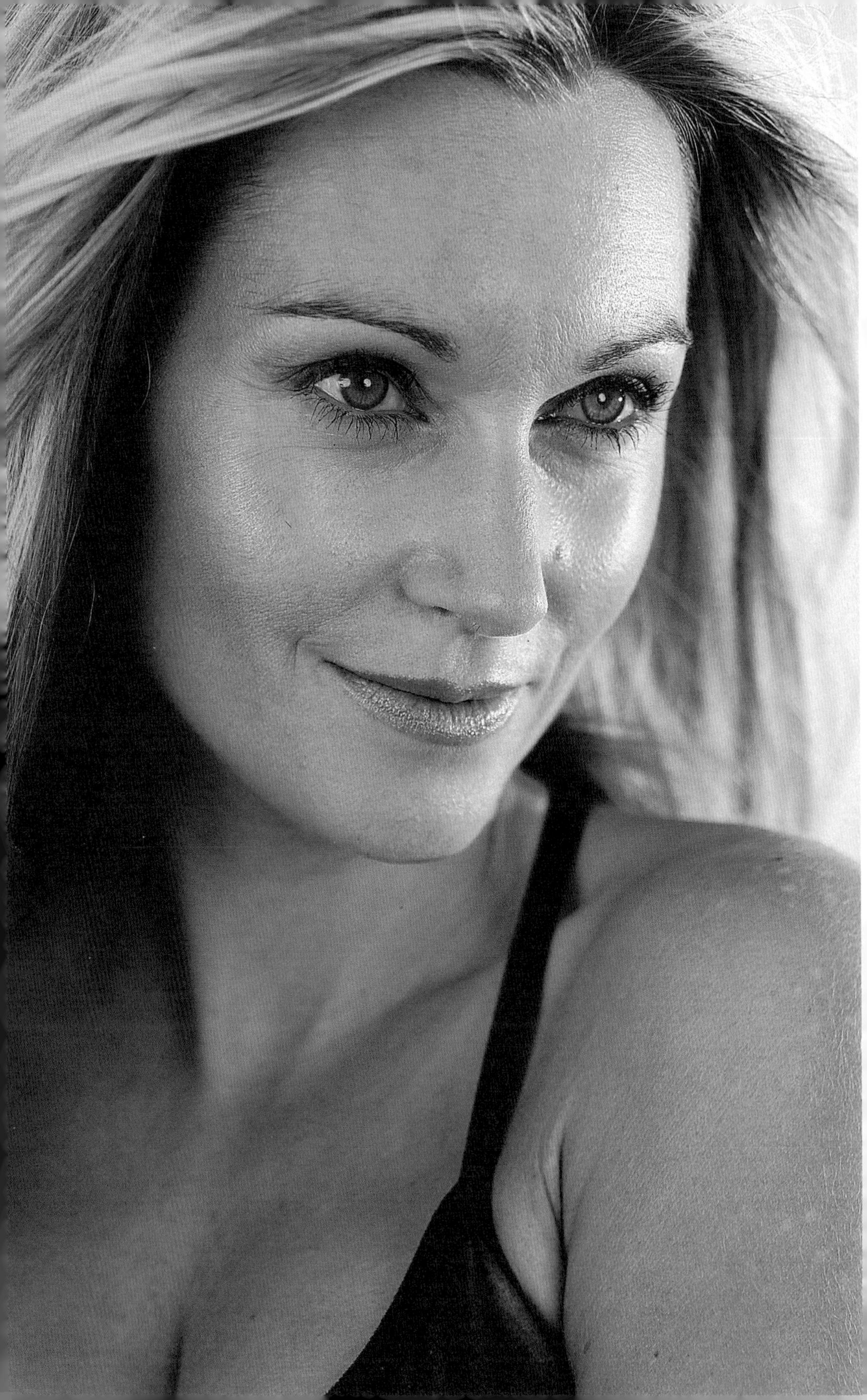

About the Author

NikkiFitness, Nicole Glor, is a regular fitness expert on Fox and Friends, and the star of 7 fitness DVDs including ***Hard Core Abs DVD, Fit Travel Workout DVD, Booty Camp, Red Carpet Runway Workout, Military Wife Workout, Baby Bootie Camp, and the Beach Bride Destination Wedding Workout*** (Amazon). She is also an AFAA certified NYC personal trainer, group fitness instructor at Crunch in Manhattan, a 200 RYT YogaFit/Yoga Alliance trained yoga instructor, author of the upcoming book "Slimnastics", a fitness columnist for Military.com and a spokesperson for SilverSport antibacterial fitness products. Her "Slimnastics" workouts focus on multitasking toning and cardio intervals to cut workout time in half and boost metabolism. Nikki's workouts have been featured in over 100 national media outlets. Get her newsletters, music playlists, video demos and DVDs at www.nikkifitness.com Search for "NikkiFitness" on Facebook and Twitter!

"Most workouts are either too easy. If they are challenging enough, they take too much time and require too much equipment. Nikki uses interesting gymnastics-inspired yoga moves with hard core cardio in just 30-minutes. It hurts so good!"

– Olympic Gymnist

"You'll never get bored – the changing scenery and different music playlists ALMOST make you forget how hard the workout is!"

– Pilates Style Magazine

Acknowledgements

This book is dedicated to my husband Jeff Glor, who writes amazing stories each day as a national TV anchor and for always telling me to be a champion, and my toddler, Jack, who is my own little personal trainer.

Special thanks to my parents, Carole and Stan Glab for always making me run around outside when I was little, for putting me through an amazing journalism school (Syracuse University's Newhouse School gave me the skills to create fitness videos and produce fitness TV segments), and for providing a great workout video shooting location in Tankah, Mexico. To my sister Kim, who became a yoga instructor herself and shot my first yoga video with me, I hope your classes come alive again.

To my college cheerleading squad who made working out the most fun anyone could have.

To Shawna, my guinea pig, biggest fan and best friend.

To friends and entrepreneurs Doug and Rachael, for our board meetings. And Lou and Kelly for friendship and marketing. To Peter and Greg at Eric Mower and Associates for teaching me PR. To Olivia at CAA for her connections and advice.

To Adam Watstein at Sharpshooter Pictures for his amazing photo and video skills.

To Kafi at New York 1 and Lauren at Fox and Friends for bringing my fitness advice alive, and live.

To Ryan at Military.com for posting my blogs. Every. Single. Week. To writers at Shape, Fitness, Women's Health, Self, Prevention and Yoga Journal – the health and fitness magazines inspire me year after year.

To sales guru Tom Davis and NFL Hall of Famer Franco Harris for my first fitness spokesperson gig with SilverSport.

To AFAA and YogaFit for training and Crunch with it's cutting edge group fitness instructors (especially Bethany, Carol and

Marc) and Manhattan clientele who always force you to up your game. And to my training clients who bring it every week.

And last but not least, to George, Alan and Steve at Regan Communications and the Boston and New York teams, especially Marzi and Erin, who are the best family, publicists and friends.

Introduction

My Fitness Mantra: Work Out Because You Can!

There is a lot of talk about working out to fit into your "skinny jeans" or "catch someone's eye" as articles and news stories on fitness resolutions, celebrity workouts, new classes, and the latest fitness gadget or class saturate the media.

I want to give you another more important reason to fit in your fitness this year: because you CAN!

Every day soldiers come home permanently injured from war. Each day someone is paralyzed in a car accident. Just head out your door and you are bound to see someone who is in a wheelchair, sight-impaired, or otherwise challenged. I try to be thankful daily that I can walk, talk, and, yes, work out!

This has become even more important to me after working with military families and having my baby. Emergency C-section surgery left me with an infected incision, and numb foot and leg from the epidural. It lasted for two months. At the time, I thought of the days when I had taken working out for granted, and now how I wished I could do 15 fifteen jumping jacks or run a mile. I had to undergo daily tests, daily nurse visits to my home, exams, and painful shock nerve therapy.

This is nothing compared to the physical and mental challenges that injured soldiers, athletes, accident victims, and otherwise impaired people go through. I thought, "If I am to get my feeling back through physical therapy, I resolve to never take working out for granted, never ditch a run because of rain, never complain about teaching a cardio-sculpt class when I would rather be at a movie."

The feeling is back in my leg and I never miss a workout. I challenge you to think that way as you read this book.

I once read a great quote in a *Prevention* magazine article by Michael Segell: "Take care of yourself, because life is a gift that can be rescinded at any time...to live irresponsibly is to dishonor that gift."

So instead of eating poorly, complaining about the gym, or skipping that workout video because you are "tired," instead live responsibly, honor your gift of health, and work out because you can and for those who wish they could!

Fitness—fit it in.

Nikki

Part 1

Chapter 1

NikkiFitness Slimnastics: X-treme New Workout

Every week as a fitness writer for Military.com, I cover new combo workouts on the market. Dance with martial arts, Pilates with rollerblading, even boots that go "boing." Then there are extreme workouts that separate the body parts so drastically that one day is pull-ups only, the next day fifty ways to do a push-up, and so on so that it takes a week to get a full-body workout in.

But you shouldn't have to quit your job to spend all that time working out, combine things that don't go together, or buy gimmicky equipment! So I decided to design my own no-equipment combo workout that is extreme without being ridiculous. I combined training from my college cheerleading and gymnastics days with favorite strengthening yoga poses and vinyasas, then added my intense NYC-style boot-camp fitness class favorites and personal training results-based moves.

Yoga meets cheerleading meets boot camp!

The NikkiFitness "Slimnastics" Workout is an athletic routine that gets you ripped in a radical new way:

- Warm up and ready your body with a yoga-based sun salute—but keep your sneakers on, you are going to need them!
- Slim and tone your legs while melting away fat and cellulite with gymnastics/cheerleading-inspired explosive plyometric cardio drills.
- Alternate the intense cardio intervals with upper body and core-cutting balance moves from gymnastics and yoga.
- Finish off in a yoga-based stretch and cool-down for the mind and body.

A word about plyometrics...

Plyometric workouts incorporate fast leaping, jumping, or skipping, basically level-change moves that require strength and power. What's more, plyo moves burn calories and build lean muscle fast.

This type of workout is especially effective for basketball and football players, dancers, runners, fitness-class enthusiasts, or anyone who enjoys activities that require jumping and landing. They build power for the jump and keep your joints, muscles, tendons, tissues, and ligaments strong and adaptable to avoid injury when you land.

I love to incorporate what I call "plyo-power" moves in my classes and fitness videos because:

- They build muscle (like simple squats) and give you a cardio workout (like jumping jacks) in just one move instead of two.
- They are more fun than strength training on gym machines.
- They cause you to explode into the move and shock your muscles to tone up faster.
- They work you harder to fight plateaus.
- They make sports activities easier and safer to perform and increase your ability to go faster and jump higher.
- They include jumping and level-change power moves that are great bone builders.

Because plyometrics are so powerful, they should be treated as an advanced workout move. If you're new to working out or recovering from injury, stick to machine workouts that isolate one muscle group first, then get into free weights and moves that require balance. Then, add upper and lower body together (multitasking toning) with cardio intervals before going to plyometrics. Plyo moves require balance, coordination, and flexibility and should be performed on a fairly soft substance as opposed to concrete.

As with other advanced exercises, your muscles need to recover, so be sure to get proper rest and nutrition, and don't do too many per week. I like to do plyometrics about two times a week along with multitasking toning workouts, cardio endurance, cardio intervals, and yoga. Plyometrics make a great addition to a well-rounded cross-training regimen.

You'll see plyometrics cardio intervals after every few body balancing and toning yoga/gymnastics poses in the Slimnastics workout.

Chapter 2

Motivation: It Starts Today

Slimnastics is primarily for those in pretty good shape. But what if you have not had a really great workout since your high school sports days and don't consider yourself someone who should be seen walking around a gym, let alone as an athlete?

If for years other things have taken priority over your workouts, and you've found comfort in fatty, sugary, and fried foods; if walking from the car to the grocery store puts you out of breath and produces enough sweat to warrant a shower; if you are unhappy with your fitness level then Part 1 of this book is for you—because that was yesterday!

Today you can change all that. It is in your power to choose any day, any minute, any reason to become a "person who works out." You can choose to change your identity to someone who has a healthy diet, who has tons of energy, and who is a role model for others who envy your drive and athleticism. You can look good in everything you try on and crave that "workout high" more than an ice cream or French fries.

You can be a person who gives exercise advice to your friends and family and who gains new workout buddies from your fitness classes. You can wake up early before the rest of the house to do fitness DVDs during the week.

This is who you will become, and it starts today. You can change who you are, starting with your mind, at this very minute. You have the power to decide what you are going to eat at your next meal and to decide to fit in some fitness today. You have the power to detox your kitchen and get grocery products that will reduce your medical bills in the future.

This is who you are, even if you are the only one who knows it now.

Make up your mind and get back a little bit of that person you might have been in high school. Day by day, choice by choice, others will see who you have become—a healthy, powerful person.

It only takes one day to change your life. I promise.

Incentives to Get Fit When You Need Them Most

Sometimes the incentives of a longer, thinner, stronger, healthier life are not enough to motivate you to get to the gym, read fitness books, or do that workout DVD. It happens to everyone. Don't despair—I am here to help.

Other important reasons to work out include increasing your performance at work (most successful CEOs are gym rats—see the office tear-out sheet at the end of this chapter).

Exercise also takes the stress knots out of your back and shoulders from a day at the computer and gives you time to think. I have gotten the best ideas and sorted out the toughest problems while jogging or lifting weights.

And speaking of the computer, exercise puts the social back in social networking. You can step away from the computer and go instead to the Thursday night fitness class, the half marathon, or your regular Saturday morning yoga studio session where you can meet new friends in the competitors, classmates, and yogis on the mat next to you, as well as the staff, salespeople, class instructors, or hottie trainers. Even home DVDs can give you an online friendship with the instructors via their facebook pages and fitness newsletters.

At home, fitness helps increase your sex drive. Increased circulation is one reason, but fitness also gives you what I call an "attitude adjustment"—you are less likely to be yelling at the hubby after a workout! Plus, an exercise routine wakes you up and gives you energy, like a coffee substitute! You'll gain more confidence, and why shouldn't you be confident when you're happy, energized, and your body looks great? A daily workout makes you want to eat better and take care of yourself in other ways, like craving a salad and water after a workout instead of wine and cheese.

So...you can have more fun, wake up, solve your problems, and de-stress. It's all in your power, so take control and put on those sneakers!

Top 15 NikkiFit Tips Special Tear-Out Sheet

Tear out this page of the book and stick it in your workout clothes drawer, gym bag, or maybe even on the fridge for some other incentives to get your sweat on!

1. Set goals that are realistic and specific. Have a set time period as your goal to help you stick to a new fitness regime. Write down your plan of action for every day, week, and so on. Start with a plan that you think you can accomplish or exceed. For example, walk for 30 minutes and then run for 20 minutes. See how many times you have to stop and walk each time. Eventually, work up to running for 30 minutes.
2. Identify and eliminate your barriers to exercise and eating well. Make a plan to conquer and avoid those specific barriers. Take each barrier or excuse and write down ways you can solve the problem.
3. Put one sneaker in front of the other. Many of us waste too much time saying we need to work out but dreading the process. Get dressed to work out and don't think about the next step. If you take it one step at a time, before you know it you will be finishing the cool-down and feeling amazing.
4. Make yourself an upbeat iPod playlist or CD. You can dance around as you clean up at home. Or you can find a hip-hop or African dance class at the gym, learn to belly dance at an adult education class or at the Y, or just plan

a girls' night out dancing. You can find a great music list on my website.

5. Make dates to see friends and family and do something that doesn't involve eating and drinking. Walk through the park, go biking in summer, ice skate or cross-country ski in winter, walk the mall, take a yoga or cardio class, or run on a treadmill right next to your friend.
6. Think of food as a fuel, not as a gift. Pass on food that is high in fat and sugar and take half the portion everyone else heaps onto their plates. If you go out to eat, you should pack up half the food on your plate in a doggy bag.
7. Practice good habits when you eat out. If you have to be at a restaurant, identify the three healthiest things on the menu and pick between those.
8. Follow the food pyramid (now the "plate") daily. Focus on whole grains, fruits, vegetables, lean protein, and calcium, not sweets and fats.
9. Don't eat any junk food lying around the office. Bring healthy sweet or salty snacks to your desk, such as whole wheat crackers, almonds, grapes, or chocolate soy milk. Buy a slow cooker so that you can prepare a healthy meal in the mornings that is ready for you when you get home (it's like having a personal chef at home all day and gives you that extra hour for exercise).
10. Drink no more than two alcoholic beverages at parties and events (if necessary, cut extra drinks with spritzers) and have a snack before these events so you don't attack the buffet line.
11. Drive less and walk more. Take the stairs when possible and never go a day without some exercise.
12. Invest in a gym membership if you don't have one already—and use it. If you don't have the money right now, buy an inexpensive workout DVD.
13. Weigh yourself everyday to remember your goals and feel good about the choices you made yesterday.
14. Keep reading health and fitness columns online. Subscribe to weekly e-mailed fitness tips for regular inspiration and subscribe to fitness magazines. Whether it's a new and healthy dish you can make, news about a recent medical

study, interesting moves to try at home, or another person's story about how he or she reached a goal—any inspiration will help. You can get my weekly tips emailed by visiting www.nikkifitness.com.

15. Pass this advice along. I saw a quote once that said, "You are the average of the five people you hang out with the most." So get your friends to subscribe to a fitness newsletter, such as the NikkiFitness newsletter, and find a partner to work out with and help you make healthy choices at a restaurant.

Working Out Helps at Work! Special Tear-Out Sheet

Tear this sheet out and post it at your workspace.

It's hard to focus on getting in shape while slouching at the computer, travelling to meetings while constantly checking your cell phone for texts and emails, and tending to growing to-do lists and stress. But you'll do better at work by adding some playtime.

By playing, I mean taking that morning bike ride, jogging in the park at lunch, going to Pilates or a cardio-sculpt class after work, and taking active vacations on your weekends such as hiking or yoga retreats.

Decide if today at LUNCH you can do any of the following:

- walk
- jog
- bike
- take an express class at the gym
- do light yoga stretches
- fill in the blank:__________

Or if you can really focus and get the most work done today with the least amount of distractions so that you can leave early or on time and...

AFTER WORK commit to one of these:

- hitting the weight room
- working with a personal trainer
- going to Pilates class
- jogging in the park
- _____ exercise with the family

You can also make a MORNING plan so that you get to bed early without a post-work cocktail:

- set the alarm for earlier than usual
- make the morning coffee and lunch before going to bed
- prepare your work outfit for the next day
- put your sneakers, keys, wallet, fitness dvd, workout book, or gym pass near the bed
- go to sleep in fitness clothes so you can make your morning workout happen

6:00 a.m.: Have to prepare the kids for their day and then do errands and chores all morning? Instead of being sluggish and holding onto your coffee cup for dear life, working out can leave you looking forward to crossing chores off your list and excited about how many calories you'll burn running around.

7:00 a.m.: Depending on where you live, you could be racing through the subway late for a meeting, sitting in traffic, rushing in from the parking lot, or organizing the kids early in the morning to get out the door. If you are deconditioned, you'll probably be sweaty, stressed, and/or too winded to say hello to the people you are doing that business lunch with. If you are in shape, you will be energized!

9:00 a.m.: Early morning presentation? If you are used to that 6:00 a.m. spin class, this speech will be a breeze to get through—with less hills to climb!

Noon: People who walk around town or the park during lunch feel less ragged and overworked during this mental and physical mini-vacation each day and can turn back on full throttle when they return to their desk. Some of the best work ideas have come to me while running around the reservoir track in Central Park, and you'll be happier with the endorphins pumping, completing your day with a smile.

3:00 p.m.: Big meeting at the end of the day but feeling the 3:00 p.m. slump? If you are not fit, coffee may be the only thing that gets you through the day, still half in a fog. But instead of dehydrating on caffeine, a lunchtime walk will have you more focused and give you time to think quietly and plan your talking points. If you are a stay-at-home mom or dad, you won't feel sluggish and wish for a 3:00 nap if you are used to pumping iron at 5:00.

6:00 p.m.: At the end of the day your back muscles may be tight with stress and your head pounding with all the work you still have on your desk. Taking a class at the gym will have you saying, "What work?"

11:00 p.m.: Up at night trying to sleep but thinking about what you need to accomplish in the office or at home tomorrow? If you jogged during the day, you'll be sleepy with a clear mind and better rested when you awake to tackle your tasks.

More exercise = better sleep = better work day.

And let's face it, the better the work-day is, the more likely we are to get promoted and be in a position to negotiate more vacation days for more play!

Attitude Adjustment

I was watching *Oprah*. I tuned in because she had a show about women's health. Most of it featured women who had trouble sleeping, a low sex drive, depression, and who popped too many prescription pills. They all admitted they didn't eat well and didn't exercise enough.

"Hello!," I yelled from the couch. Why didn't they realize that eating right and exercising are the most important things you do all day?

Many of us need an attitude adjustment. Here are five ways to do it:

1. **Change your priorities**. There is a comic strip that I love of a doctor asking a patient why he doesn't exercise. The patient says he doesn't have a free hour in the day. The doctor asks, "Do you have twenty-four hours a day to be dead?"
2. **Eat to live—food is a fuel not a reward**. We discussed some of these issues in a recent wellness seminar held at my alma mater Syracuse University. Emme, a plus-size supermodel and women's advocate joined in, and we discussed how

to strive to be happy and healthy, instead of just thin. Many people make the mistake of thinking of food as a gift, our one pleasure for the day. In reality, it's simply a fuel to keep us living and moving. We are supposed to eat in order to move—and move a lot. Food fights diseases and keeps us strong, if we have a good relationship with it.

3. ***"Work out because you can!"*** As I mentioned earlier in the book, this was a fitness mantra I came up with when I lost the use of my leg for several months due to a botched C-section. Be thankful you can use your body, that you are not injured or disabled. Instead of moving a lot, we tend to work hard for everyone else and sit at a desk or in the car most of the day then collapse on the couch. No wonder we are depressed, overweight, and sick. We need an attitude adjustment in food and fitness. Working out gives me the sense of satisfaction I crave from that fatty dish or second glass of wine. Being active stops me from yelling at my husband. It works like caffeine to wake me up yet helps me sleep like a log. It prevents injuries. Studies show that exercise and eating right can get you off of many medications. People who exercise crave bad food and alcohol less often. They are nicer to be around.
4. **Don't procrastinate.** You can't control what happened yesterday or last year, but you can control what you do today: *"If you went running when you first thought of it, you'd be done by now!"* Get outside or put on that fitness DVD. Why put your health off until tomorrow when you might be too sick to do anything at all by then? In the military, you know that life is too precious to waste. The best thing you can do all day is turn off *Oprah*, put down the soda, and go for a jog on your way to the health food store.
5. **Find positive influences.** "*You are a combination of the five people you hang out with the most.*" I saw this quote in a NYC bathroom, but it is so true. Surround yourself with people who put an emphasis on happiness, health, love, and fitness. You can also find them online through social media or in fitness magazines. For more diet and exercise tips and information on workout DVDs, visit www.nikkifitness.com. E-mail your fitness questions to nikki@nikkifitness.com.

Chapter 3

Shape-Up Instructions

It's time to check in with your body.

Did you spend the entire winter hibernating? Splurge too much on summer vacation foods? It is never too late to get a spring back in your step and get in shape. Here's how to start!

For the novice, do safe **Level 1 Moves:**

Duration: One of the best ways to start a workout is to start slow and isolate muscle groups with toning workouts for the whole body for 45 minutes every other day, or for just the upper body for 30 minutes and another day do lower body for 30 minutes—and steady state cardio for as long as you can every other day or every third day for the first two to four weeks, four to six times a week.

The moves: Muscle toning should be done every other day to let muscles recover. If you have access to a gym, focus on isolating machines. For example, a seated shoulder press machine, a seated abductor/adductor thigh machine, and many others allow you to sit and just work one area of the body. This will keep your workout safe and start to build muscles before attempting standing balance challenges and multitasking toning moves (see Level 3). If you are working out from home, start with seated arm moves using light barbells (seated bicep curls, for example) then standing squats and lunges holding onto a wall. Kneeling push-ups also work several areas of the arms and the core, so work on doing them every other day and gradually increasing the number of reps. Do regular crunches, side-lying oblique crunches, and cross crunches and spinal extensions for the lower and upper back.

For cardio: Start with walking or jogging for 10 minutes, then work up to jogging for 20 minutes. If you prefer an elliptical or a bike, slowly start increasing your duration and speed. You can do cardio on the days you don't do toning or do both on the same days if you have the energy.

Duration: Do cardio for 30 to 40 minutes every other day, and do combo muscle workouts for 30 to 60 minutes every other day, four to six days a week.

For someone who may have hibernated a little too much this past year but used to work out in the past, your muscles have memory so you can start at Level 2.

Level 2 Moves

Once stronger, a novice can increase the weight amount and move on to combo moves that work the upper and lower body together. If you are a moderate exerciser, you can start at this level and skip level one. At level 2, you can get rid of the gym machines and do multitasking toning moves and increase the weight. These include plie squats with overhead shoulder presses, lunges with biceps curls, calf raises with tricep overhead presses, bent-over glute leg lifts with upper back rows, and full push-ups. Work the lower back with Supermans and add more complicated abdominal moves. Start with a weight of around five to eight pounds with eight reps. Once you can do fifteen reps easily, then increase the weight to ten to twelve to fifteen pounds and go back to eight to ten reps. Once you get to fifteen reps with ten to fifteen pounds, move onto to Level 3. For more on these moves visit the website for the free newsletter or fitness DVDs.

Level 3 Moves

This level combines muscle and cardio in intervals and gives harder combo moves but cuts the workout time to just 30 minutes (this is the level featured in my other workout DVDs). You do your multitasking toning moves with balance challenges for 3 minutes followed by 3-minute plyometric cardio intervals (see interval section) where you go medium effort for the first minute, hard effort for the second minute, then recover with medium to easy effort on the third minute. Because these moves are intense and the transitions are fast, you burn more calories and up the metabolism.

Duration: You'll get your booty camp workouts with muscle and cardio on the same day, then on alternate days you can also add cross training classes like dance, yoga, Pilates, spinning, swimming, and long runs/road races because your body will be ready to take on more and more challenges. Work out six days a week...and you'll be ready for Slimnastics!

Train to Improve Your Push-up Power

One of the most common questions I get from readers at Military.com, class members, and training clients (especially women) is about building up strength to do full strong push-ups—and you'll need them for Slimnastics. I have training clients who tell me they can't do two push-ups on their knees. Once we start the steps below, I have them doing 100 to 150 full push-ups (on their toes) during each hour-long session! They can defend themselves and have great-looking arms.

So many women have trouble building up the strength or just say they hate doing them and give up. It's very important for women to have strong upper body strength. Just follow these steps:

1. Start standing an arm's length away from a wall and count how many you can do against it. If you can do more than twenty, move on to the next step. If not, practice every other day until you can do twenty against the wall, trying to do one or two more each day. (You need to give yourself a day to recover in between.) Finish by stretching your chest muscles: link your fingers behind you, lift your arms upwards, and hold for 15 seconds.

2. Find a table, couch, weight bench, bed, or counter. This should be around knee- to waist-level high. Stand back far enough so that you can lean your body diagonally onto the bench, holding yourself up with your arms. Do the push-ups at this level, working slowly up to twenty at a time, practicing every other day. Bring your chest down to the bench or whatever you are practicing on and be sure to focus on keeping a straight line from your ankles to your hips to your shoulders. Hands should be farther than shoulder-width apart. Keep the body aligned and don't hinge at the hips. It's better to only do one perfect move rather than ten reps with poor form. Watch yourself sideways in a mirror or have a friend watch you and tell you if your hips tilt up to the sky or you let the belly sink to the floor instead.
3. Move to a step (either a step from an exercise class or a step at home on a staircase). Start on your knees with feet together. Again, focus on your form being a straight line from your knees to hips to shoulders while bringing your chest and chin to the step and work your way up to twenty.
4. Now you are ready to do them on your feet, still on a step. Ankles, hips, and shoulders in line, chest and chin to the step.
5. Congrats! You are ready to try the full push-up. Once you work up to twenty, you can start trying to do more...

My Secret 100 Push-up Arm and Ab Workout!

In a 30-minute workout, do ten full push-ups. Turn over and do 60 seconds of regular crunches. Flip back over and do ten push-ups. Repeat this push-up/1-minute abs routine ten times, and you've just done 100 push-ups and toned your arms, chest, and core.

Also, you can brag to your friends about how many you can do instead of hiding the fact that you can't do any!

Trainer's Tip: Work the opposing muscles. You should always work your upper back muscles—the opposing muscle group—to avoid a muscle imbalance. An imbalance will cause the shoulders to round forward, the pectoral muscles to tighten, the trapezius and rhomboids to be overstretched, and other back conditions to develop, even pain. You can strengthen your back by doing weighted dead rows, weighted reverse flies, or by lying on the floor, arms out to the side away from body at shoulder level to form a T, and lifting the chest and arms off the floor. Squeeze the shoulder blades towards each other and release down for twenty reps.

For more back routines, see the next section.

Back Up Your Health

Imagine a virus going around that causes pain and stops you from driving, picking up your toddler, shopping for groceries, and exercising.

Now imagine a medicine that prevents this virus. You would take it, right?

This pretend "virus" is back injury. It is real and happens to people every day when they trip and try to catch their balance, roll out of bed, bend over to pick up a bag, take a kickboxing class, or perform a dead lift. The medicine I prescribe to avoid "catching" the virus is a combination of a few exercises for the upper and lower back. I will explain two easy ones here today.

Lower for Living

Strengthening your lower back muscles is important for people who don't exercise on a regular basis, but it is equally important for those who do exercise but overlook the lower back. If you have a bad lower back, you can't do those crunches, bicep curls, lunges, or daily living activities.

Upper for Posture

The upper back exercises are important as well, especially if you sit at a computer or hunched over a desk much of the time. It is equally important if your exercise routine includes push-ups and bench presses but not exercises that work the opposite muscle group—the trapezius and rhomboids. Hunched posture can cause painful knots and strains, increase chiropractor bills, and give the wrong first impression.

Moves

Airplane: This exercise will work both the upper and lower back. The airplane (pictured below) is performed by lying on your stomach with arms extended out to the sides at shoulder level.

1. Lift your head, chest, arms, knees, and feet off the floor, leaving just your torso on the mat. It is also important to keep looking at the floor, not cranking your head up to look at the wall in front of you. Keeping your gaze on the floor keeps the neck in line with the spine. Hold for 3 seconds and release. Repeat ten times.
2. Next, speed up the move to fifteen faster singles, not pausing at the top.
3. Finally, hold the arms, legs, and chest up to the top of the move, keep the legs and chest lifted, and "flap your wings" by moving the hands up and down for ten repetitions. As a bonus, this exercise also tones your tush!
4. Stretch. That completes one set. When done with each set, do a cat stretch on all fours and drop the head while rounding the back up to the ceiling.

Balance Reach: To perform the balance reach, stay on all fours on hands and knees. Keep looking at the floor as you reach your left leg up and straight behind you, lifting your right arm straight in front of you. Hold the leg and arm up for a count of three and release. Straighten and lift your right leg and light arm simultaneously, hold for three and release to complete one repetition. Continue to gaze at the floor throughout the move. Do ten reps for one set and finish with a cat stretch.

Back it Up!: Before I became a trainer I didn't realize the importance of working my back as much as working my abs. I highly recommend that you add these moves to each workout you do. Take this advice from someone who went through a back injury and could not do normal daily tasks. In Slimnastics, I will do more challenging back exercises like wheel push-ups. Work up to doing them and...take your medicine.

Ten Plank Variations for Perfect Core Toning

Planks are one of the cheapest, easiest, and quickest ways to tone your body anywhere you go. They work your abs all over, and if you get creative you can also add glutes, thighs, triceps, shoulders, upper back, and pecs to the list! Here are some of my favorite plank variations (from my *Fit Travel Workout*) for your next sweat session.

Note: When I mention a regular plank position, I mean balancing on your elbows (forearms) or hands (the top of a push-up) and toes, facing the floor, with hips in line with the shoulders and knees and hands or elbows directly under shoulders. Look in front of your hands to keep neck in line with spine. You'll look like a perfectly straight plank parallel to the floor, lifting the belly button towards the spine. In a side plank you will balance on one arm and face the side of the room instead of the floor.

1. **Forearm Plank Hold:** Balance on your forearms and toes, hold this for 30 seconds, and work up to 3 minutes!
2. **Push-Up Plank (pictured):** Do a push-up, then turn to the right, balancing the weight on your left hand, opening your right hand to the sky, and staggering or stacking the right foot on top of the inside of the left as you balance on the outside of the left foot. Come back to a full plank, do a push-up, and then repeat on the other side.
3. **Plank Knee Cross:** Hold a regular plank and then balance on your left foot and bring your right knee under you towards your left elbow. Keep your hips low to the ground. Return to full plank and repeat on other side. Make it harder by taping the opposite hand to the foot or by "can-canning" the leg—after you bring the knee toward the opposite elbow, straighten the knee and kick the leg out toward the left. Bend it again and return to start.
4. **Outer Thigh Side Plank:** Plank on your right hand or forearm and lift your left straight leg off the right leg and toward the sky. Lower leg and repeat ten times. Move into a plank on the other side and repeat. Make it harder by bending your lower leg and holding a weight in your top hand. Straighten the arm to the sky as you lift the top leg. As you lower the leg, lower the hand and weight behind your neck, keeping the elbow pointing to the sky the whole time to work the triceps in a half French press.
5. **Glute Plank:** Balance on your hands or forearms and lift your left straight leg off the floor. Move it over the right foot and then return to start. Repeat on that side ten times and then switch to the right leg lift and cross. Make it harder by bending the left leg at ninety degrees with the sole of your

foot facing the sky. Lift and lower in pulsing motion for ten reps. Repeat on the other side.

6. **Hip Taps:** Get into a side plank on your left forearm. Lift hips off the floor and then lower them to tap the left hip to the floor and lift again. This works your obliques in an extreme way if you do twenty or more! Repeat on the other side.
7. **Thread the Needle:** Get into a side forearm or full side plank on your right arm. Lift left arm to the sky and stagger the feet so the top (left) leg is in front. Sweep your left (top) arm toward the mat and "thread" it under your right armpit, reaching for the back of the mat while rotating your hips to face the ground and balancing on your toes. Rotate your body back to a side plank and repeat fifteen times then do the same on the other side.
8. **Plank Crunch:** Hit the obliques again by getting into a full plank on your left hand and stagger your feet with the bottom (left) foot in front this time. Bend your right elbow and put your hand behind your head. By balancing on your right (top) foot, bring your left knee across to your right elbow to "crunch" then return to start. Repeat fifteen times and then switch sides.
9. **Spiderman Plank:** Get into a full plank on your forearms or hands. Balance on your right toes as you bend your left knee out to the left and towards your left elbow. Return to start and repeat twenty times, then do the other side.
10. **Upper Back Plank Rows:** Get into a full plank position with medium weights under your hands. Lift the right elbow to the sky and return to the ground. Repeat on the other side. Do twenty reps switching arms each time. Wrists hurt? Instead of balancing on weights, you can also work the upper back by doing down dog planks or dolphin planks. Start in a plank on your forearms or hands and then push hips to the sky and push hands into the mat like you are trying to rip it in half between your feet and hands, Your biceps should be next to your ears. Return to start and repeat twenty times.

BONUS Reverse Plank Stretch: Get some relief from your hard work and sit on the floor with your hands on the floor next to your hips, fingers pointing towards feet. Your knees should be bent and feet flat on the floor. Push into your hands and lift your hips off the floor, letting your neck be an extension of your spine and looking at the ceiling. This stretches the chest and shoulders while toning the core, glutes, and quads.

Next time crunches make you crazy, fight the plateau with this plank series!

Put an "I" in Fitness with Interval Training

If life is too busy for you to remember what days to do strength training and which to do cardio, or if your metabolism is slowing down and you really want the most out of your workout, say "I." "I" is for "interval."

Interval training can come in different forms, such as alternating jogging and sprinting when you run in the park, for example. But what I do at Crunch Fitness in Manhattan and in my fitness DVDs is take this a step further. By combining fast and slow cardio with multitasking muscle moves in one workout, you will not have to worry about doing legs one day, arms the next, and cardio the third. You really do get everything in one workout, and six very special benefits as well:

1. **Appetite:** Recent studies in the *Journal of Sports Science and Medicine* show that subjects who did cardio and muscle toning intervals ate over 500 less calories per day after four months than those who did cardio one day and all muscle toning the next. They say the combination can cause a change in hormones that control your hunger.
2. **Stress:** The same study showed that being active reduces cortisol levels that are caused by stress.
3. **Endurance:** In biking or "ride" classes, the study showed that short high-intensity sessions, sprinkled with recovery instead of steady state pace, boosted endurance.
4. **Metabolism:** With interval cardio and muscle training sessions, you can also get the benefits of increased metabolism. If you up the intensity of the workout through alternating cardio and muscle moves, you increase excess post-exercise oxygen consumption. This is what we trainers call "after burn." Resistance training builds metabolism-boosting muscle while cardio makes the fat over the muscle disappear. Then after your workout you will

continue to burn more calories while reading, watching TV, and sleeping!

5. **Better Toning:** According to a 2008 study published in the *Journal of Strength and Conditioning Research*, women whose muscle routines only included weightlifting gained less muscle strength, added less muscle endurance, and lost less body fat compared with those who ran for a minute before each strength set.
6. **Osteoporosis Prevention:** We all know those people, women especially, who only diet and run, bike, and do cardio machines. They think skinny is better than toned, sleek, healthy, and strong. A hump on your back and broken hip doesn't look good at any age. Young women are becoming more and more prone to stress fractures because of reduced calorie intake and cardio, cardio, cardio. They don't realize that it's not about being skinny as the Olson twins, it is about looking toned and being strong for everyday life. God forbid you fall into a situation where you need physical strength to save your life, but you want to be ready for it. Lifting weights builds strong bones. Sprinkle it in to stand up straight, defend yourself, and walk without a limp. That is sexy.

So overcome workout boredom and make the hour fly by. Alternate between fast and slow cardio and multitasking muscle moves that work arms, abs, and legs at the same time. Working out is the most important thing you can do for yourself, and there should always be an "I" in fitness.

Working Out After an Injury

ACL surgery, a slipped disc, a broken arm, or knee injuries don't have to stop you from working out. Here are some tips, moves, and machines that can help you stay in shape while you heal.

Machines: I normally stay away from most of the stabilizing and isolating machines at the gym because you usually sit and only work one muscle group instead of multitasking your moves for arms, legs, and ab work. However, if you're injured, machines at the gym can be your best friend.

Cardio with a Lower-Body Injury

If you've got a lower-body injury (or are pregnant) and want a safe cardio exercise, try the arm spinner. There are many names for it including the "arm wheel" and "upper body ergometer." This looks like a padded seat with a back and a bike wheel at shoulder level. The "pedals" are actually handles. You can sit and spin in an easy resistance and go fast for intense cardio or add resistance to get your toning and cardio at once. There's also the seated cross-trainer that looks like half of a Nordic Track. You sit to stabilize your lower body and use pulleys to twist at your middle and pull the arms with resistance.

Toning with a Lower-Body Injury

Seated upper-body workout machines are ideal if you're a beginner or in rehab; otherwise, I prefer to have healthy clients workout out while standing, lunging, balancing on one leg, standing on a BOSU ball, or seated on a stability ball. The good thing about seated machines is that they isolate the area you're working, leaving the rest of your body at rest. A good circuit is a shoulder press, upper back seated pulley, assisted chin-ups, reclined chest press, lat pull down machine, seated barbell bicep curls, and a triceps barbell overhead French press. You can also invest in tubing for about ten dollars and find exercises online, including hooking tubing to a door or chair and increasing resistance by color-coded tubes.

Cardio and Toning with an Upper-Body Injury

Of course with an arm or shoulder problem, you can use the treadmill, the elliptical, the stair-stepper, or a stationary bike. Other options for toning without jarring and painful movements can include the leg press for quads and glutes, the hamstring curl, and seated inner and outer thigh (abductors and adductor) machines. Don't forget to do calf raises with a machine or freestyle. Standing squats and lunges may be okay as long as you are not in pain, and be sure to use a wall or something stable to hold onto.

Core Work with a Lower-Body Injury

If you just have an issue with putting weight on your leg, use a chair. You can hang from the seat and use your elbows to stabilize yourself. Lift the knees or leg with your abdominals without having to hook your feet under anything. Another great machine is the ab trainer where your head and hands rest in the machine so that only your core works. Legs can be on the floor or braced on the machine depending on the size and style. Additionally, if you have an upper-body injury, you still may be able to do crunches by simply folding the arms across the chest and crunching on the floor or hooking legs under an incline bench.

Warm-Up and Stretch

A good way to avoid further injury is to warm up for 5 minutes before a workout. Warm-ups include easy, slow cardio with no incline or resistance on the machines listed above or rhythmic limbering—mimicking the toning moves you're going to do later, but without weights and with music. Stretch each muscle group you worked for 20 to 30 seconds after your workout.

Resources

Ask your gym sales rep, manager, or personal trainer for recommendations or machines specific to your location or use the tubing and free weights at home to isolate areas safely. Moves from my multitasking fitness DVDs can also be broken down so you perform just the arms or just the legs parts of the routine. Physical therapists are also great resources. They'll typically nurse your injury back to health but they can also give tips on keeping your healthy muscles toned without damaging the area you are taking care of. Always consult your doctor before starting a workout routine, whether you're injured or not.

The gym can still be your playground to keep you sane, happy, and healthy while you heal.

When It Feels Like a Workout from Hell

My lungs are on fire. I can't even tell if my legs are getting tired because I am breathing so hard I can't even close my mouth. I am suddenly working above my target rate and would fail the talk test...and if I did talk, it would be to curse the treadmill! I had to cool down and do some muscle machines and yoga with the rest of my hour at the gym.

This is a personal trainer after three months away from running. Because of medical issues, I had to stop my normal five-mile runs several times a week and start from scratch. The scenario above was after only 15 minutes on the treadmill.

It made me think about how I always advise clients and readers to just get started with their daily workout and that they will feel so good during and afterward that they will be more than happy they made the effort. But that day on the treadmill I was anything but happy.

I took home two lessons with my sweat-drenched self...

1. For those struggling to get in shape for the first time: I know that, as a workout addict, it WILL get better and be worth the effort. But that is because I have seen the "promised land" of working out when you are IN shape. I couldn't wait to get back on the treadmill "horse" and get to an hour of running and feeling MORE energized, not less.
   But if you have NEVER been athletic, and don't really know how truly great it can make you feel, I sympathize. I finally remembered why so many people quit after just two weeks of trying to get into shape. It doesn't feel good at first. For those of you struggling to get into shape for the first time, trust me, it does get better and won't feel like lung and muscle torture forever!
2. Let's say you ARE in shape, but getting bored and lazy with your workout, and you think that a week or two off won't matter.
   IT DOES.

I still worked out during the end of my pregnancy and after six weeks even with my medical complications. The only thing I could not do was endurance cardio because of a numb leg from the epidural. Upon recovering, I was back almost at square one after three months away!

So DON'T take that vacation from healthy workouts—just challenge yourself and cross-train. Find a way so that you won't have an uphill battle gasping for air to fight bulge.

Soon you will turn the workout from hell into a hell of a workout!

Part 2

Chapter 4

Warm-Up: A Salute to Slimnastics

The warm-up is essential to your workout so that you don't get injured by diving in too fast. You can't do many push-ups with a pulled biceps muscle, so you'll protect future workouts and improvements if you take five minutes before you work out each day. You can also protect yourself from injury by checking with a doctor before trying this or any other workout.

Yoga-based **sun salutations** are a great way to warm up, especially if you don't have 10 minutes a day to sit on the floor and meditate. The breathing with sun salutations de-stresses you while the moves prepare your muscles for work. As they say in YogaFit teacher training, one breath = one movement.

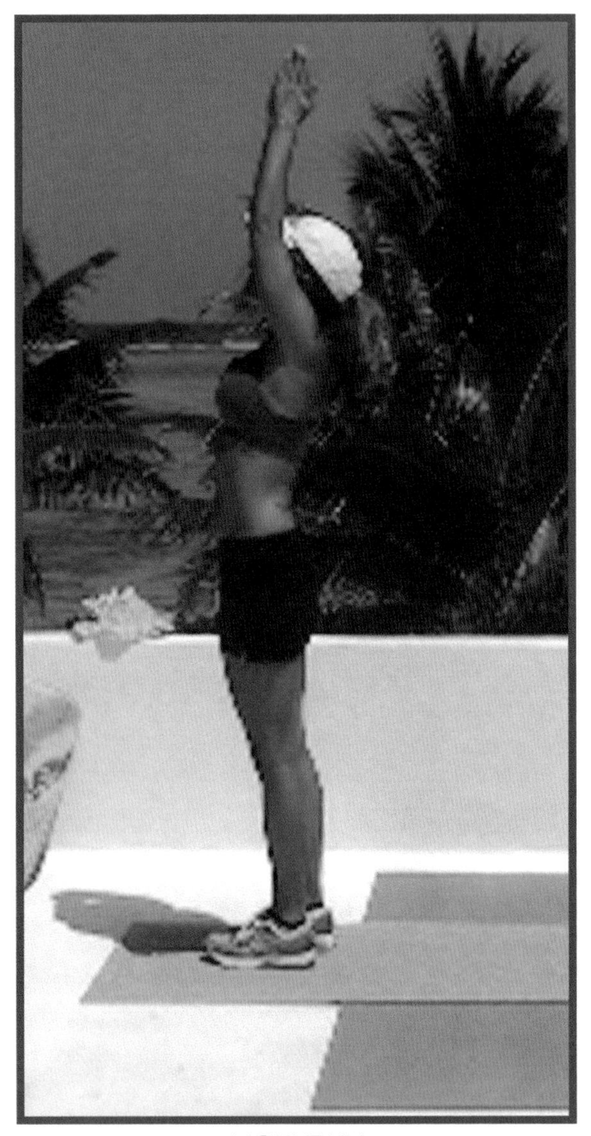

MOUNTAIN

Mountain: Begin in standing position, called mountain pose. Inhale the arms overhead, letting the palms meet in prayer, and exhale as you fold forward, hinging at the hips, sweeping arms out to the sides and down toward the earth. Keep a micro-bend in the knees for a light hamstring stretch—later you will straighten the legs for a deeper stretch when you are warm.

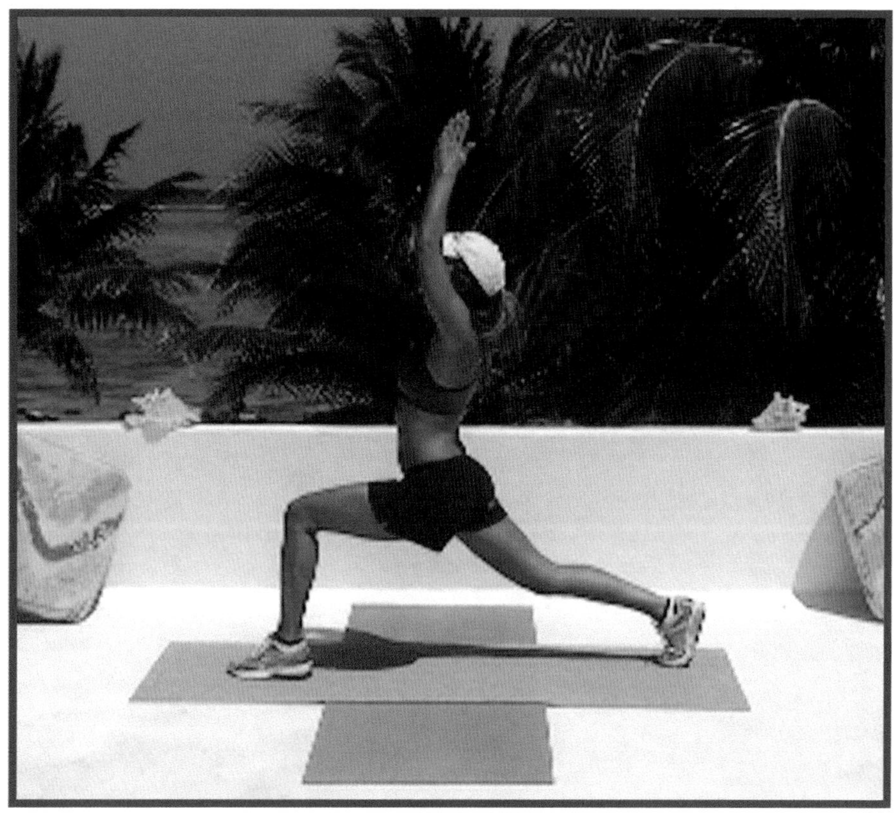

CRESENT LUNGE FULL

Lunge: Inhale while stepping the right leg back, and if it is your first time through the series, lower your right knee to the mat, slightly behind the hip. Lifting the arms toward the sky into crescent lunge, stretch up while the left knee stays bent at a ninety-degree angle.

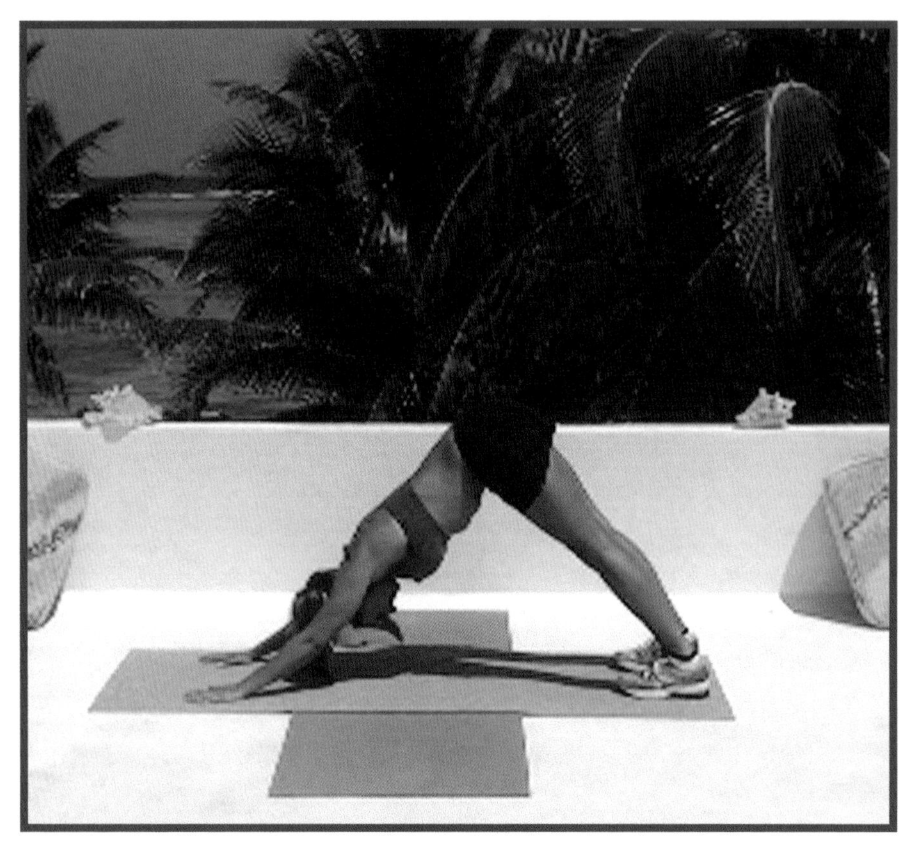

DOWN DOG

Down Dog: Exhale and place hands on either side of the left foot, then step the left foot back next to the right about hip-width apart. Using the core strength, lift hips up towards the sky in an upside-down V. Keeping the fingers wide and elbows straight, but not locked, reach the heels towards the floor but not touching. Inhale slowly and fully here while pedaling one heel closer to the floor, then bending that knee and reaching the other foot closer to the floor to wake up the calf muscles. Exhale fully and bring heels back toward the ground.

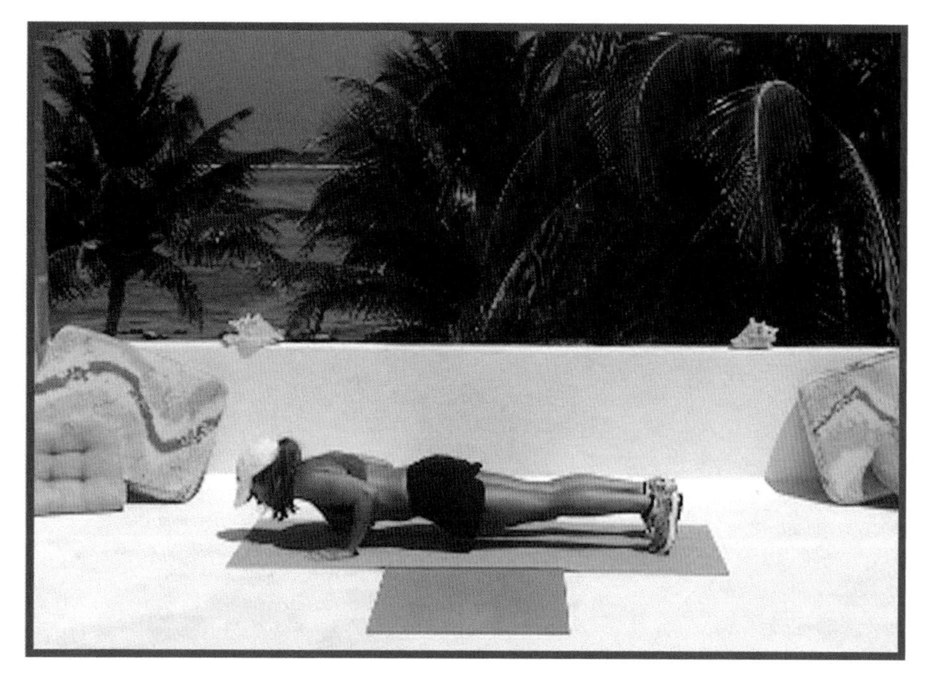

CHATURANGA

Plank/Push-up: On the next inhale, shift the weight forward into a plank, or *chaturanga dandasana* (Sanskrit). Your shoulders should be lined up directly over your wrists, abs tight, and hips in line with shoulders, parallel with the floor. If it is your first time through the series, you can lower the knees to the floor in a modified plank.

Exhale, and with elbows close to your ribs, lower down (like a triceps push-up). If it is your first time through the series, follow with cobra. If not, follow with up dog.

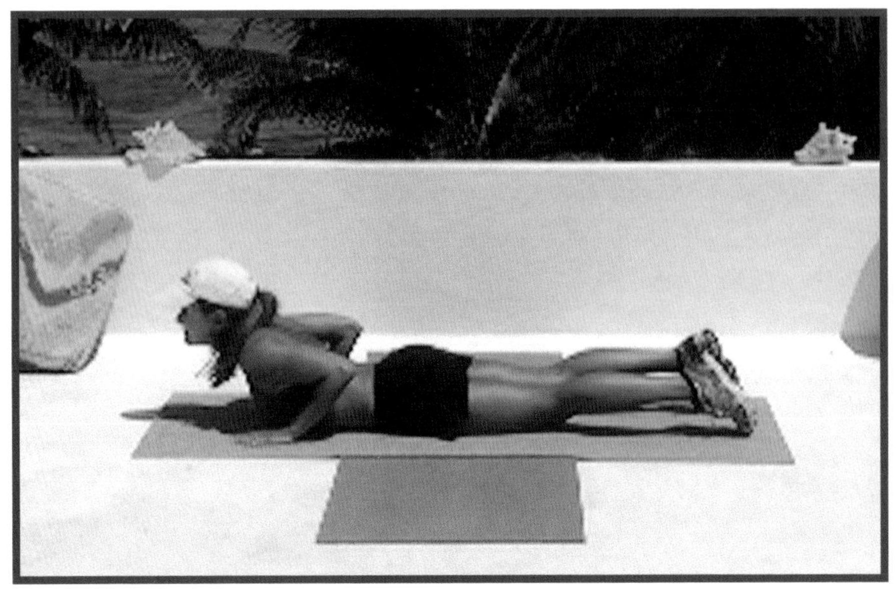

COBRA

Cobra: Keeping hands under the shoulders, rest the belly on the floor and engage the lower back muscles to lift your head, chest, and shoulders slightly off the floor. Picture a cobra with the snake belly on the floor but head lifted up. Snakes don't have hands so don't put any weight onto yours—instead use your back muscles. Inhale through the move. You can always choose cobra instead of up dog (I usually do) to add a back warm-up and strength to your workout.

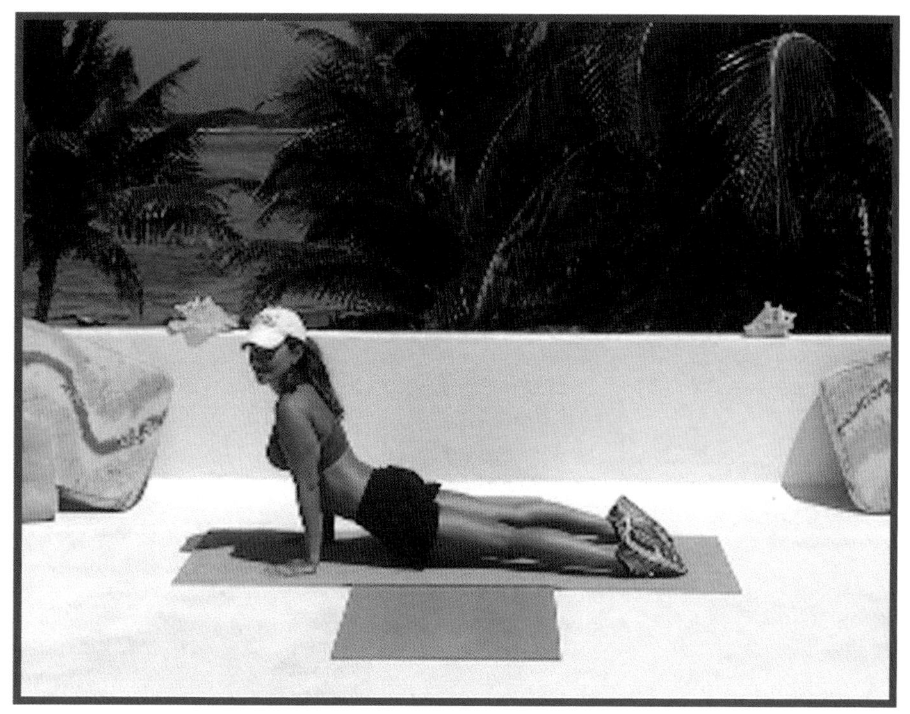

UP DOG

Up Dog: If you have done the series a few times, you can choose "up dog" for a slight backbend. From a hovering triceps push-up (*chaturanga dandasana*), keep the chest and quadriceps off the floor, flip the feet from toe balance to balancing on the tops of the feet, and push through the hands to lift the chest and head while straightening the elbows. Inhale through the move.

Exhale into down dog again, engaging the core.

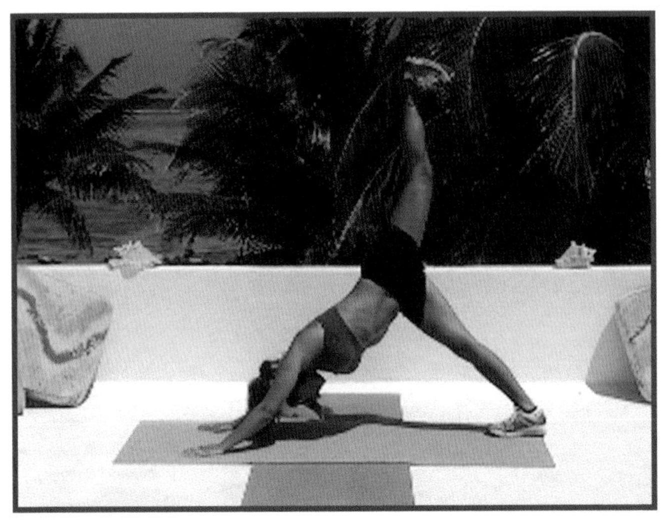

THREE LEGGED DOG

Extend the right leg high and behind you into "three-legged dog."

Lunge: Inhale and lift the hips to swing the right leg through and between the hands, keeping knee over ankle. Lower the left knee if it is your first series. Lift the hands to the sky again.

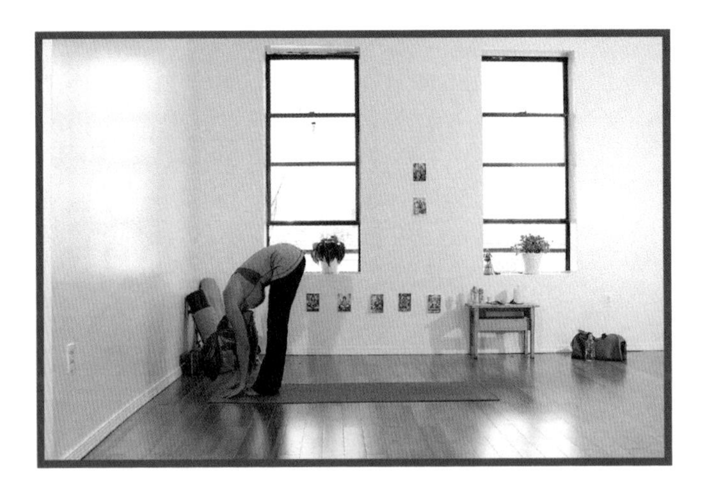

Forward Fold: Exhale the hands to the earth and step the back leg forward between the hands. Straighten the knees as much as is comfortable for another light hamstring stretch.

Mountain: Inhale and hinge at the hips, keeping back flat and sweeping the arms into a reverse swan dive to standing in mountain with hands overhead in prayer.

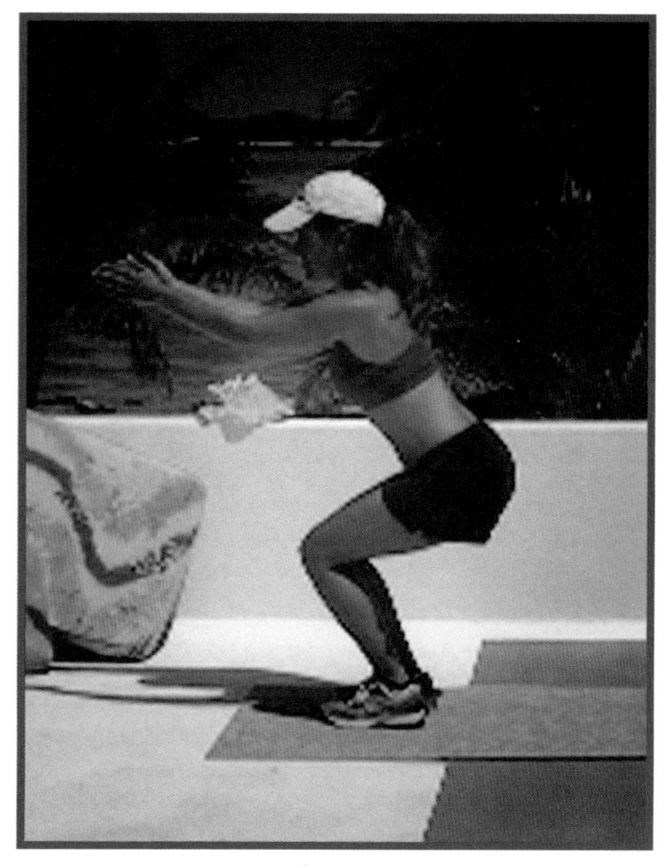

CHAIR

Chair: Exhale and lower hands to the knees or extended in front of you at shoulder level while bending the knees and sitting back into an imaginary chair to create warmth and strength in the quads and glutes.

Repeat: Inhale into mountain, exhale forward fold. Inhale, stepping back with the LEFT foot this time into crescent lunge (knee up or down). Exhale to down dog. Inhale to plank, exhale to triceps push-up hover, inhale to cobra or up-dog. Exhale into down dog and into three-legged dog with the LEFT leg. Inhale and sweep the leg through to lunge on the other side. Exhale to forward fold. Inhale to mountain, exhale into chair.

That completes your first series on the right and left. Repeat on the right and left leg four more times and you'll be prepared for a warrior workout with arms, legs, back, core, and mind warm and ready!

Chapter 5

Workout for Warriors

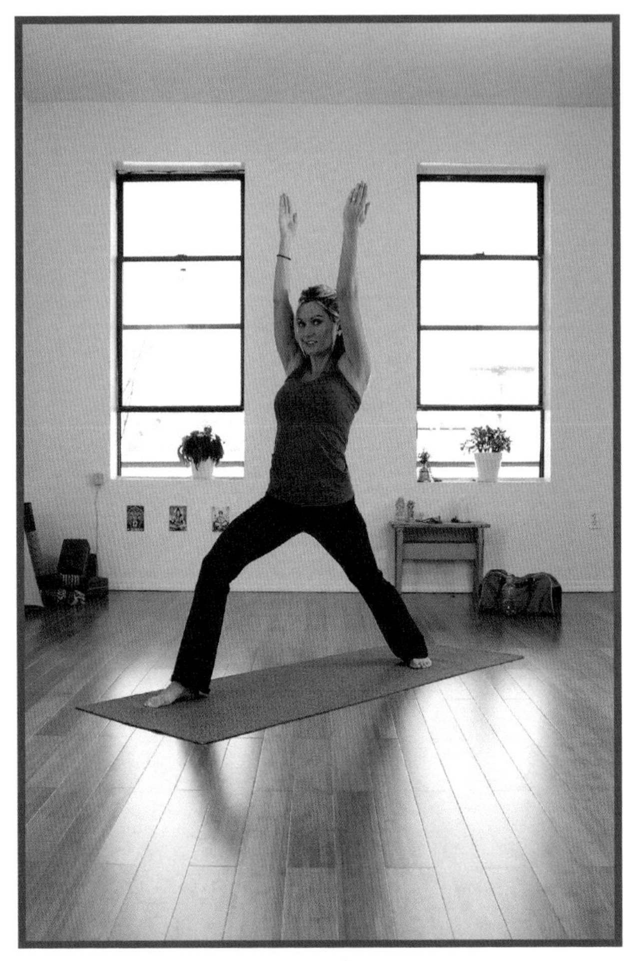

WARRIOR I

Warrior I

Stand at the front of your mat in mountain pose. Step the right leg back about the length of one of your legs. Heel is down and toes are angled forty-five degrees toward the front right corner of the mat. Bending the front left knee, the quad should ideally be parallel with the floor. Both hips are aiming at pointing straight ahead to the front of the mat as the arms reach up towards the sky. Engage both legs and push into the outside (pinky toe blade) of foot. Look toward the horizon past the front of your mat.

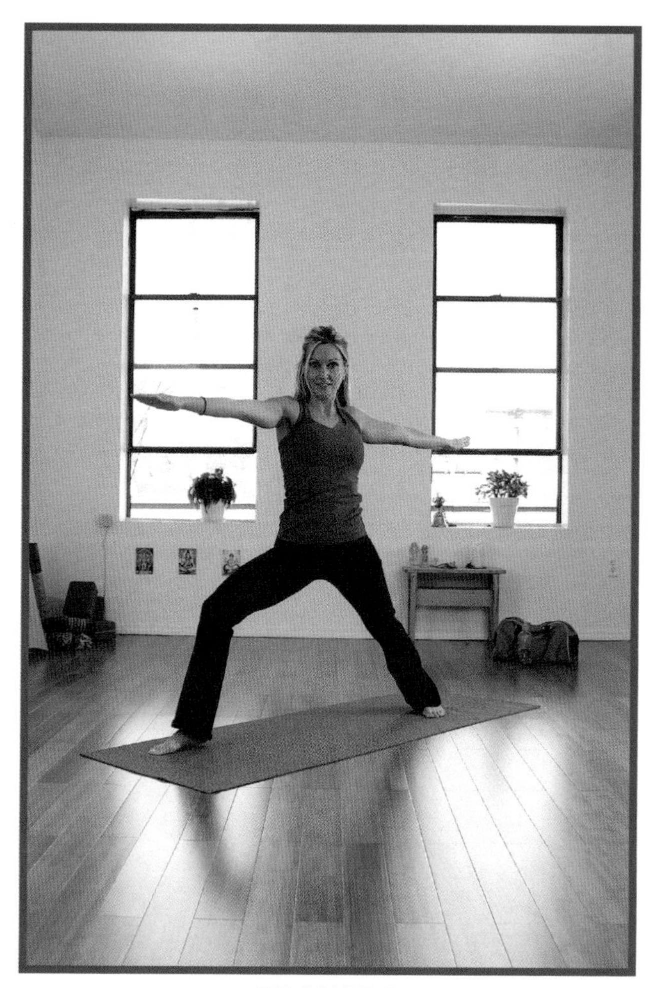

WARRIOR II

Warrior II

From warrior I, lower and open the arms to the right side of the mat while opening hips at the same time in the same direction. Arms should be at shoulder level reaching forward and back, palms facing down. Engage the left inner thigh to push the left knee back to the left corner of the mat and behind you to keep the knee over the ankle and work your muscles.

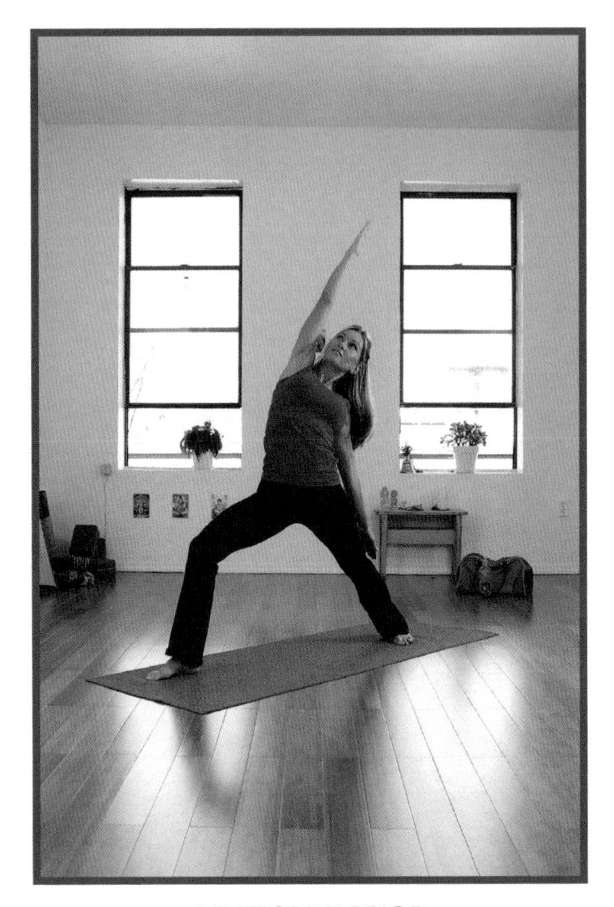

REVERSE WARRIOR

Reverse (Peaceful) Warrior

Keeping the left knee bent and quad parallel to the floor, flip the right palm up toward the sky and then raise your arm up as well so the palm now faces behind you. Lower the back right hand to gently rest on your back right thigh or allow it to float just above the leg. Enjoy the side stretch along your left ribs as you lift up through that left hand while grounding down into both feet.

Transition: Windmill the arms to frame your front foot on the mat and step back to down dog. Either perform a *vinyasa* ("flow") into plank push-up, up dog, and down dog again or move right into warrior I on the other side by sweeping right foot forward between the hands and lifting arms to the sky.

Repeat warrior I, II, and reverse warrior on the opposite side.

Cardio Interval – X Jump to Split Jumps

Stepping off the mat sets the scene for cheerleading-inspired moves like X and split jumps.

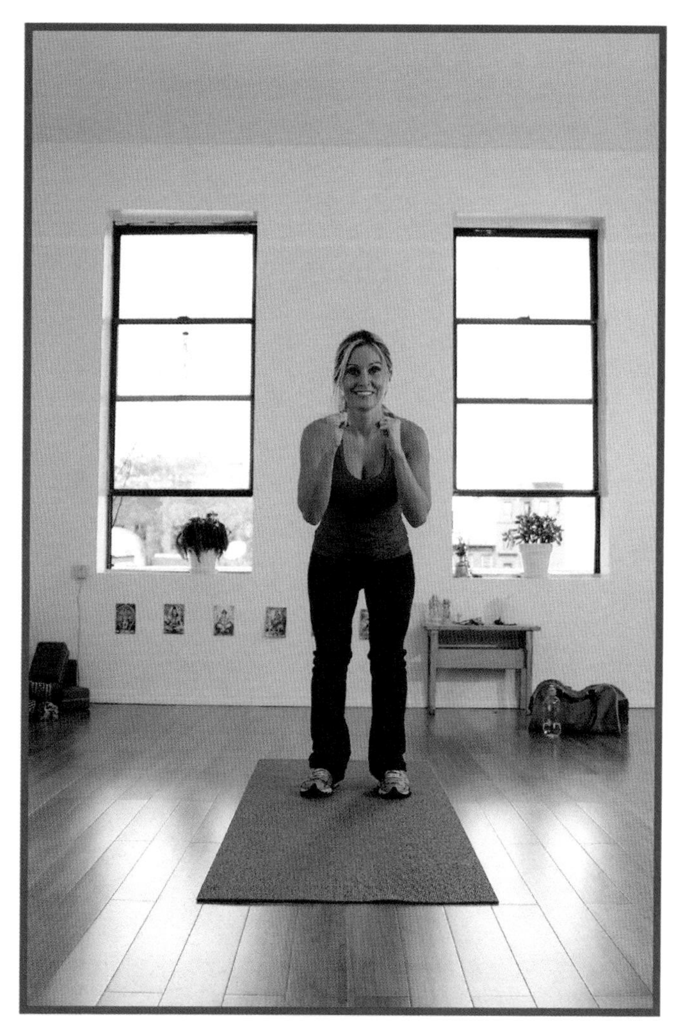

X JUMP PREP

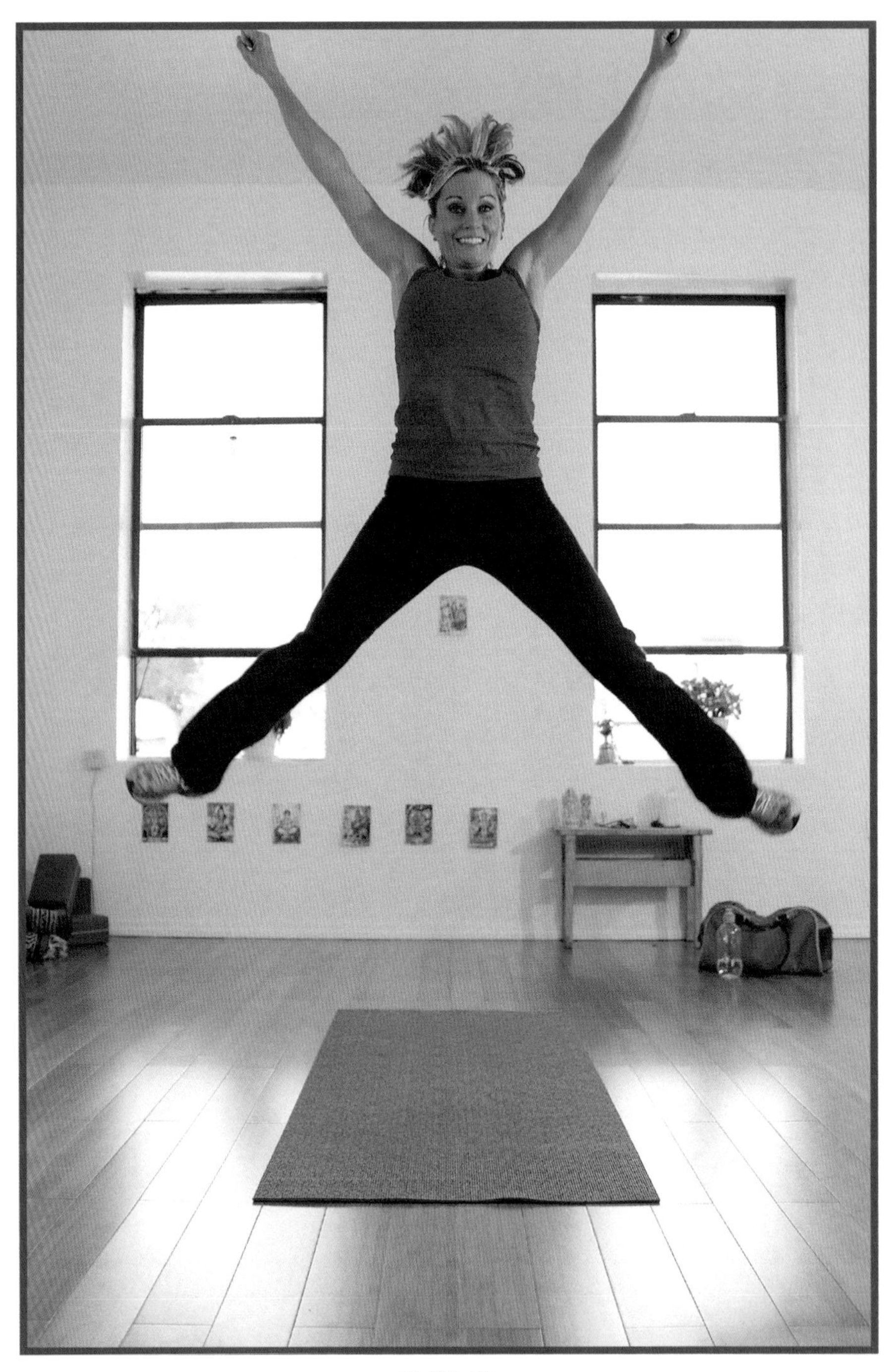

X JUMP

Perform three squats in fast succession counting one, two, three. On the "and," jump into the air using your leg muscles and punch the hands to the sky and land on four. Repeat. One (squat/stand), two (squat/stand), three (squat/stand), and jump, four (land). Make it advanced: turn the X into a toe touch (pictured).

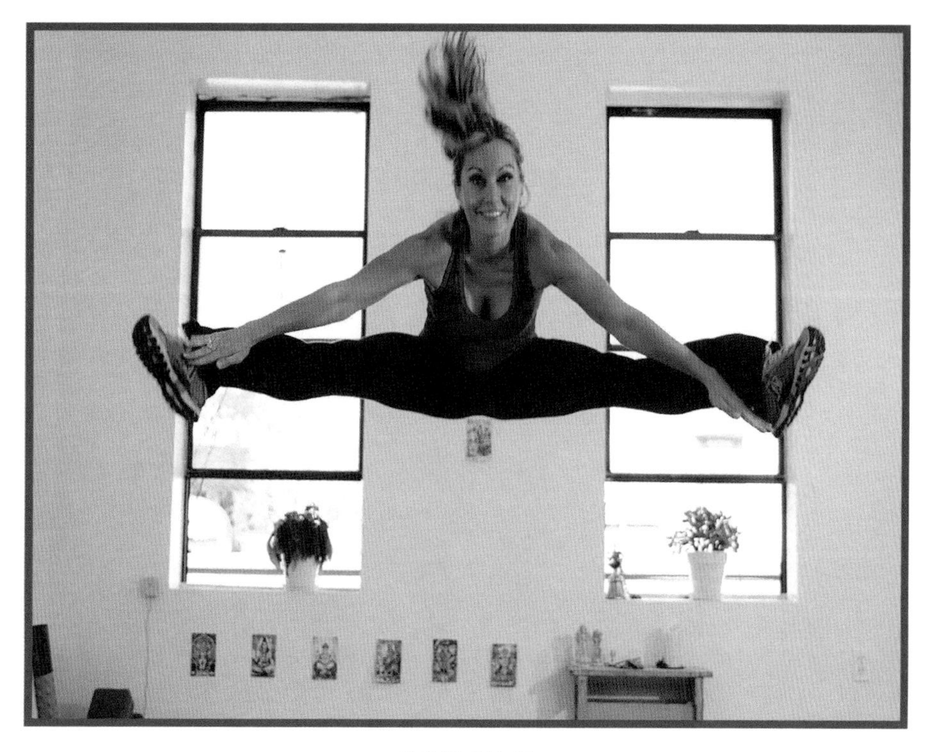

SPLIT JUMP

For the split jump, jump high into the air with arms extended overhead and legs long, like an exclamation point. Rebound on the floor and then sweep the arms in front of you for momentum. At the same time, jump and lift both legs out to the sides into a split and reach your hands for your heals.

Recover with Five Sunflowers

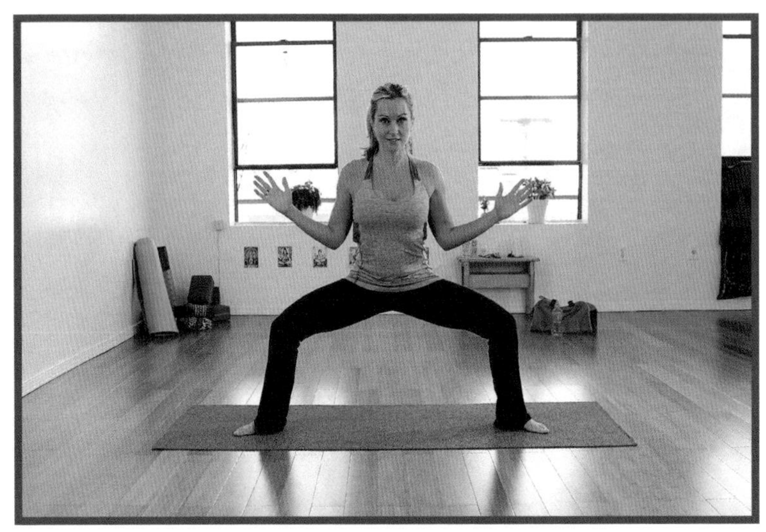

SUNFLOWER FLOW

Stand with feet wider than shoulder-width apart towards the long edge of your mat.

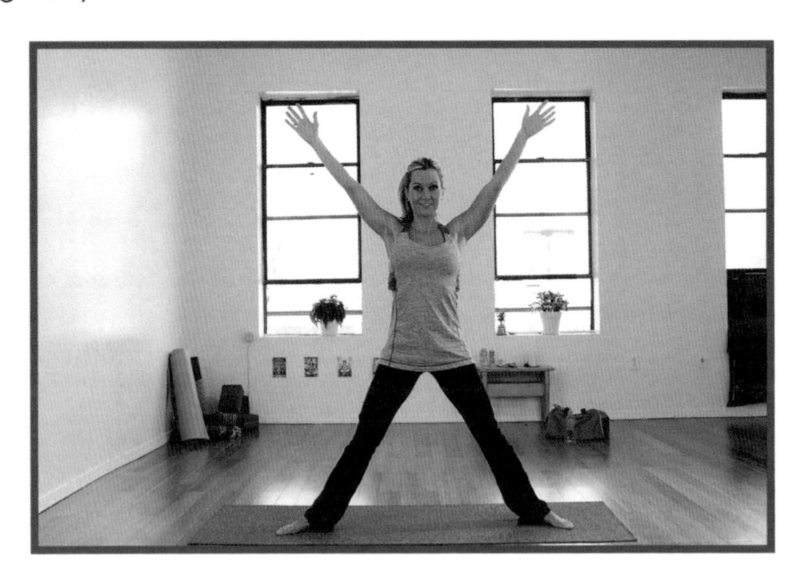

Bend the knees so that the knees line up over the ankles and open the arms out to the sides and sweep them towards the floor.

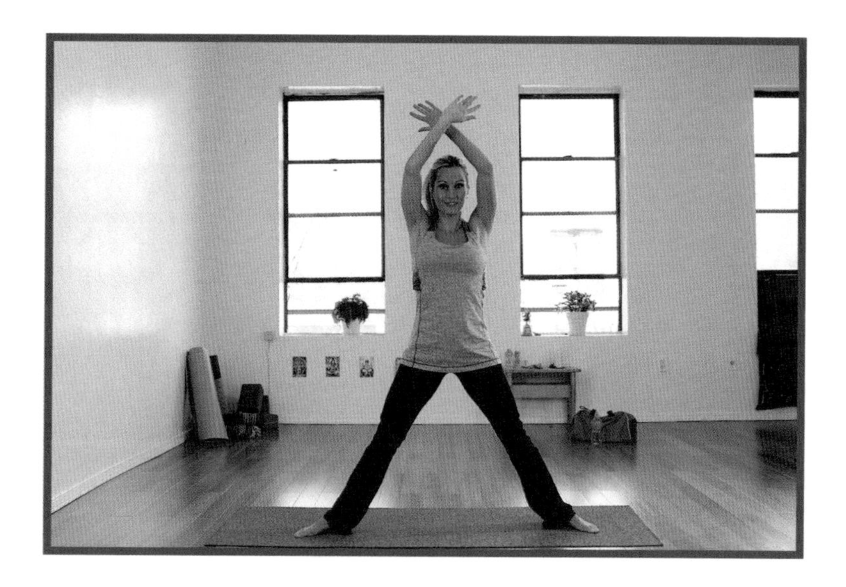

Straighten the legs to standing and sweep the arms overhead.

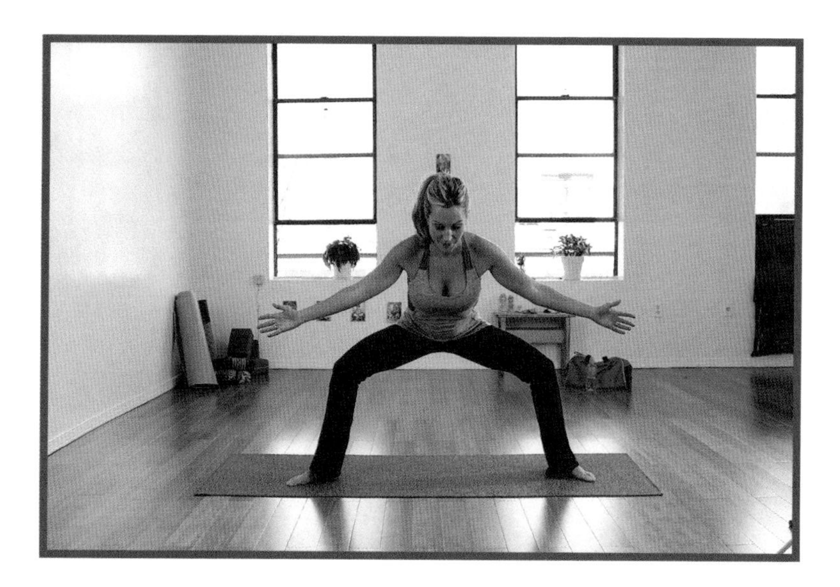

Bend knees again at ninety degrees and sweep the arms down towards the floor hinging at the hips.

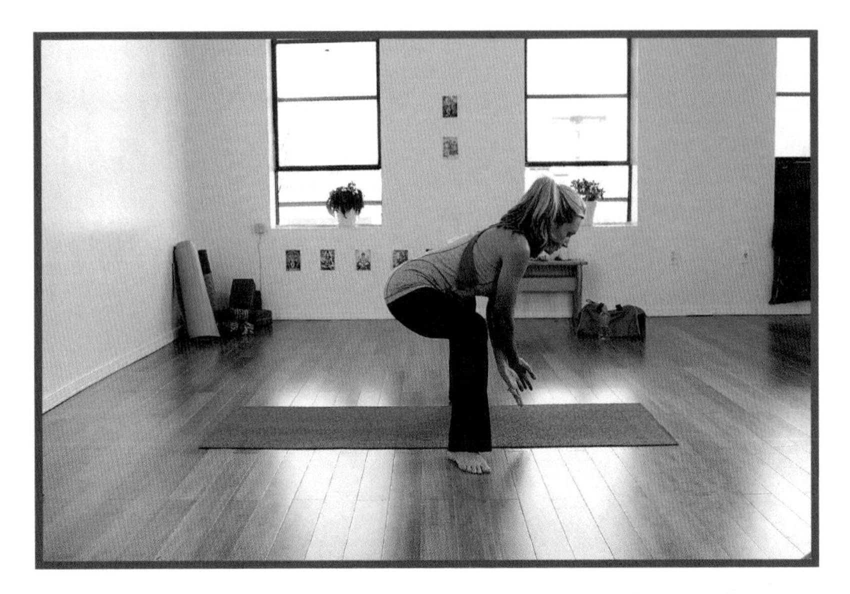

Picture your fingertips drawing the edges of a sunflower and repeat eight times to let the heart rate slow down and catch your breath.

Chapter 6

Triangle to Ta-Da!

Triangle

While still facing the long edge of the mat with feet wider than hip width, turn your right toes to the short edge of the mat and turn your left toes up to a forty-five degree angle exactly as we did before in warrior. Hinging at the hips, bring the hips back slightly and extend the arms up to shoulder level.

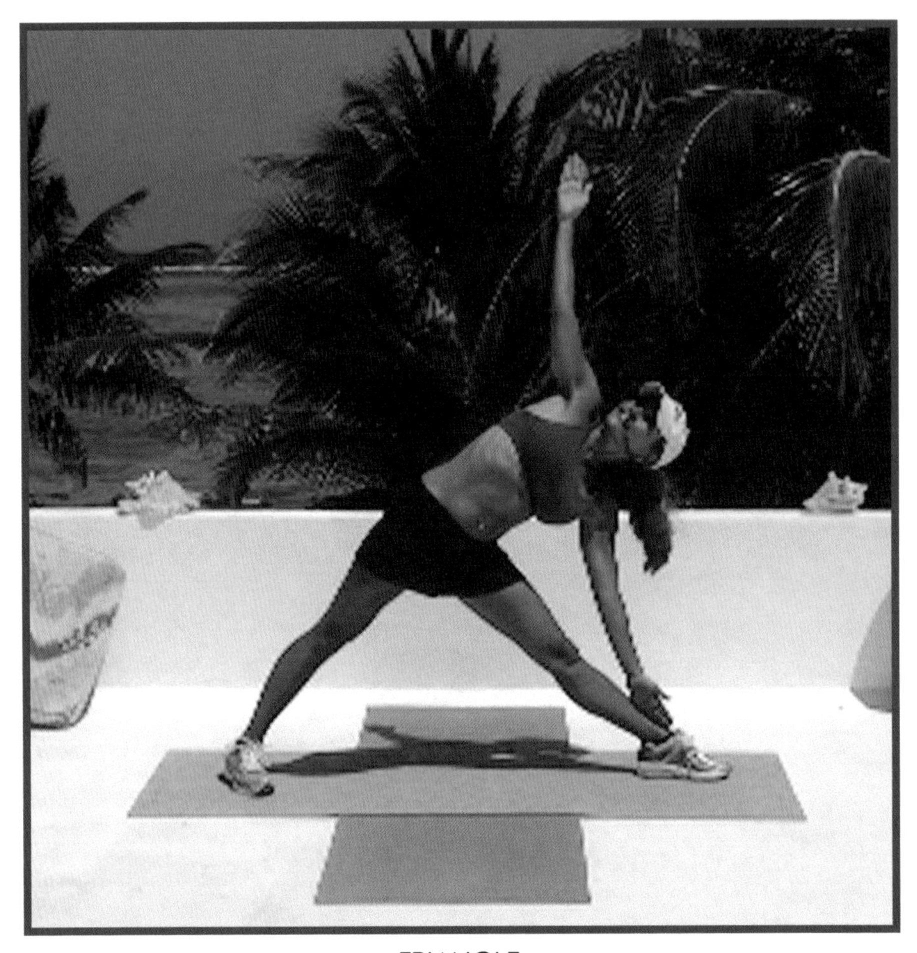

TRIANGLE

Reach the right fingertips into the "future" in front of you, and then tick-tock the hands so that the right one reaches towards the earth and the left reaches for the sky. You can use your oblique strength to dangle your right fingers over your right ankle or rest the hand onto the shin for support. Keep the entire body in one plane, as if between two panes of glass. Open up through the chest and shoulders to the front of the long mat edge and look up to the sky, keeping the neck in line with the spine and shining a light forward through the crown of the head. Breathe for three deep inhales and exhales and then reach through your top hand to come back to standing.

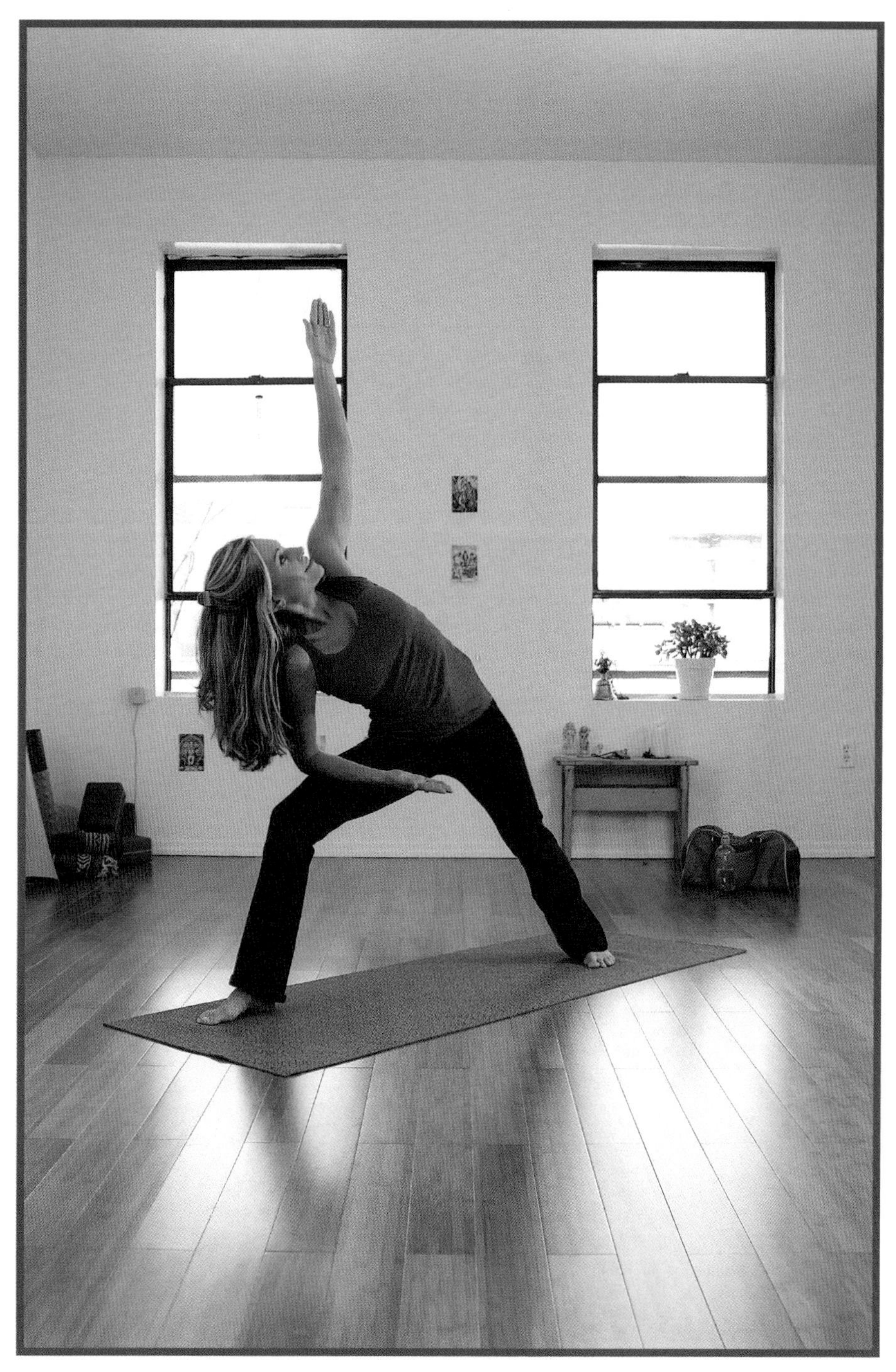

SIDE ANGLE

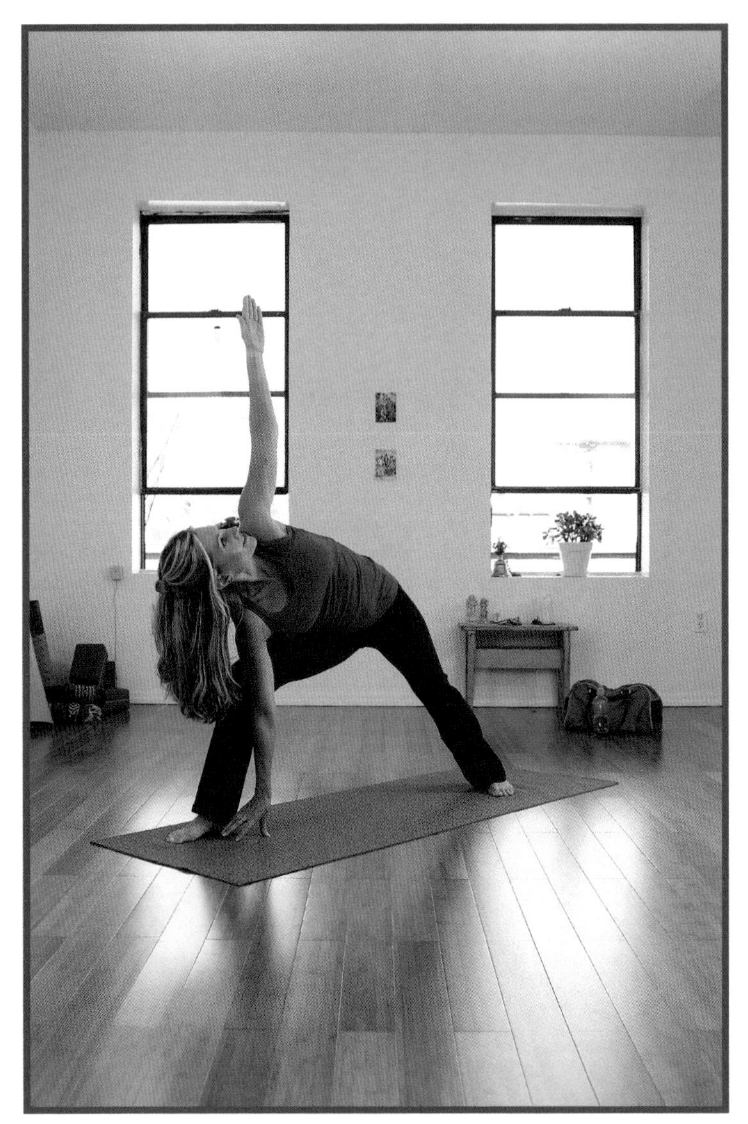

Side Angle to Bird of Paradise:

After coming up from triangle, bend the front knee into warrior II again, then bend the front arm and rest the forearm onto your front right quad, lifting the left arm to the sky again. Stay here or to go deeper you may be able to reach your right hand to the floor on the inside of your right foot. In this position the right tricep presses into the right knee and the knee presses into the arm—creating a groin and inner thigh stretch.

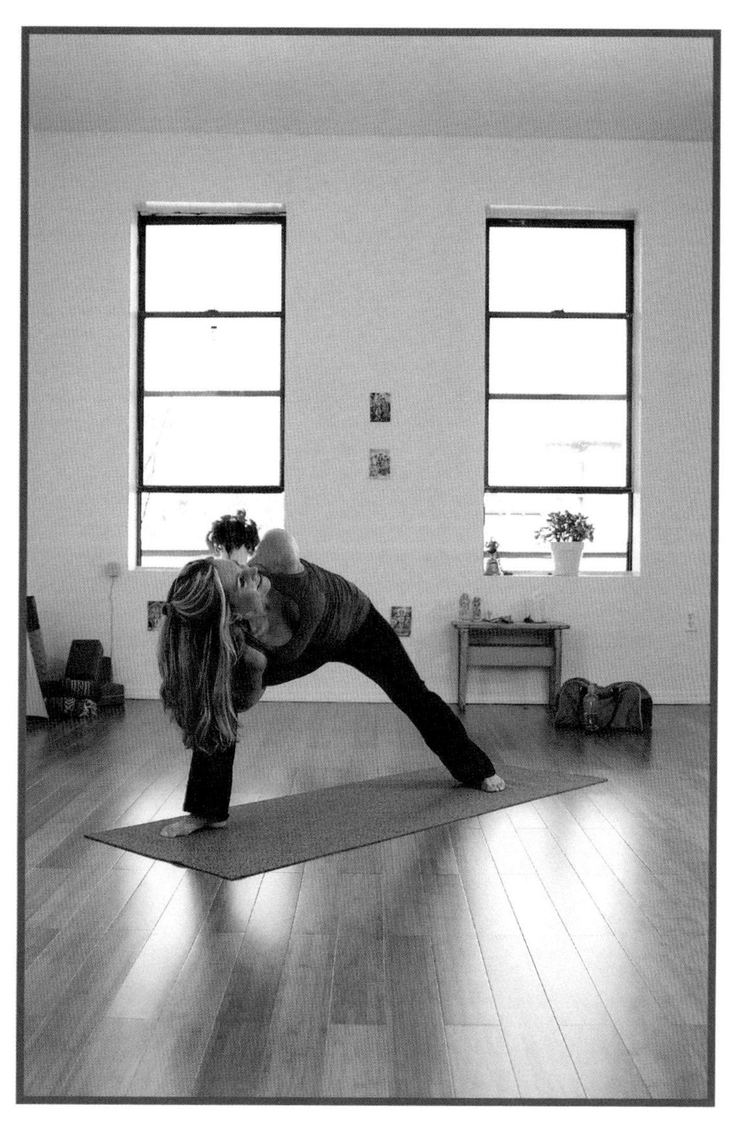

SIDE ANGLE BIND

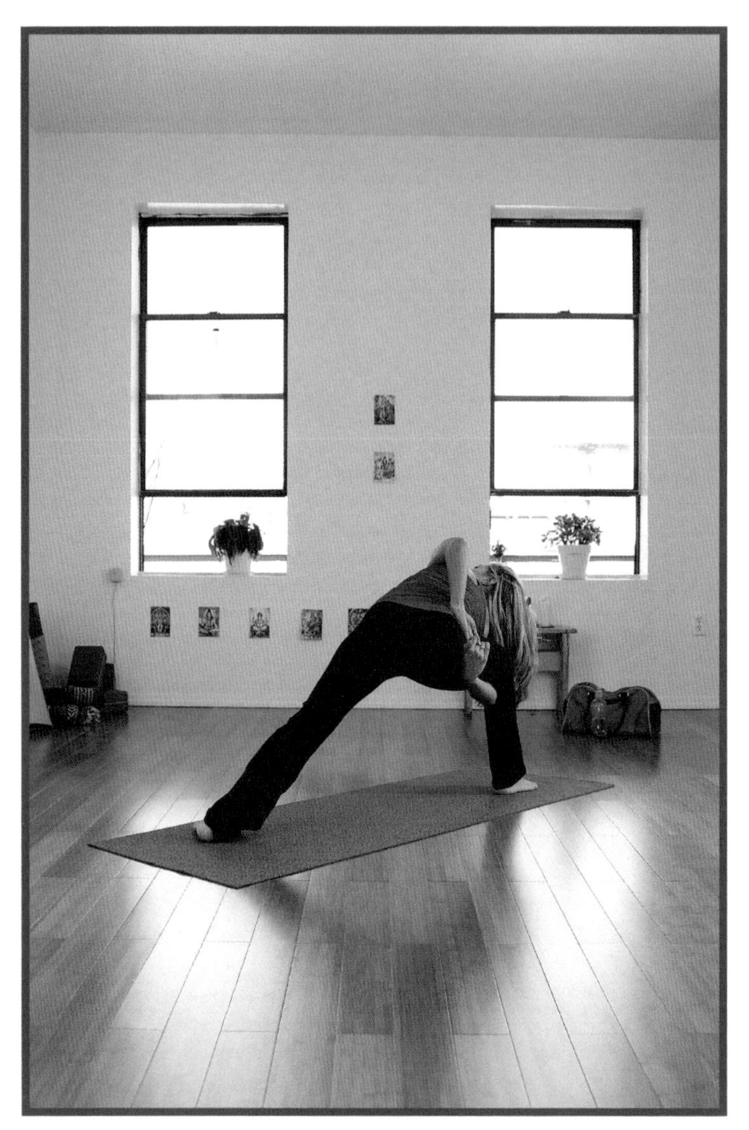

SIDE ANGLE BIND BACK VIEW

Hold for three deep breaths, then if you're feeling flexible, reach the top left hand down along your waist and the bend it behind the hips with the palm facing out. Reach your bottom right hand under the right leg to bind with the left hand and support the pose with strong legs.

To move into bird of paradise, simply step the back left leg forward a few feet and shift your weight into it.

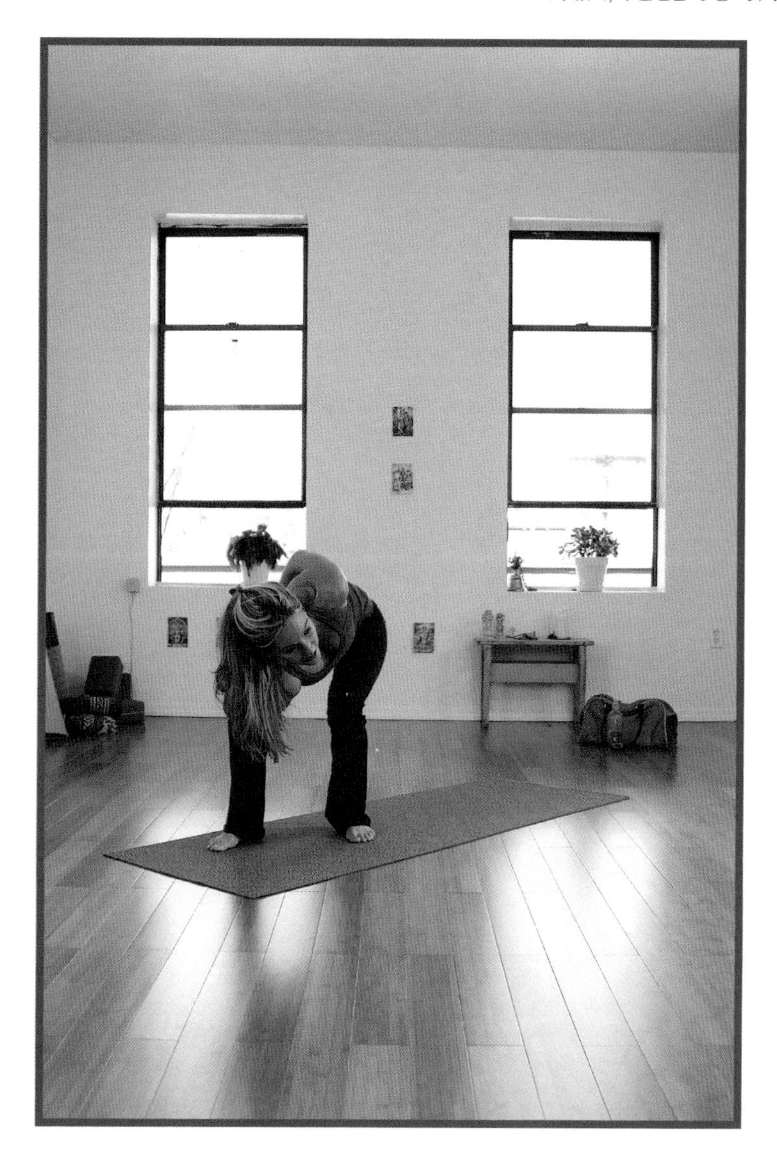

Keeping your hands in a bind, stand up and extend the right leg.

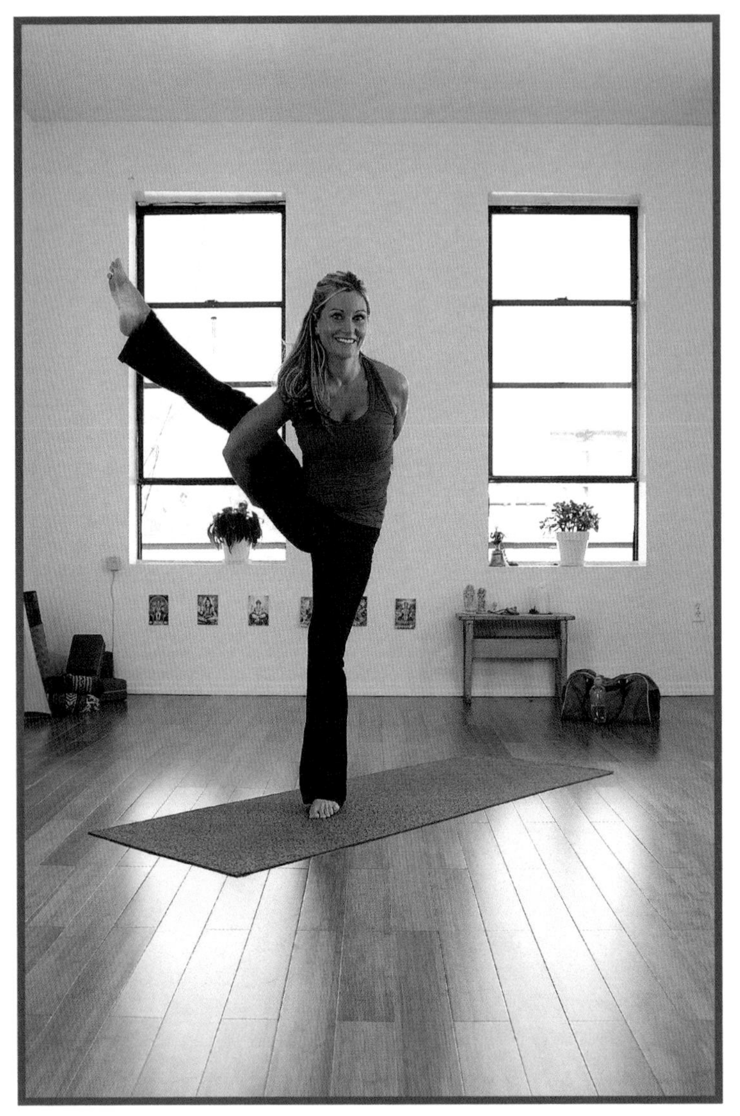

BIRD OF PARADISE

This will resemble a heel stretch but with your arms locked under the leg.

Hold for three breaths and then lower the bound leg, step the left leg back to start, unbind the hands, and come back up to standing. Face the long edge of your mat and prepare for triangle, side angle, and bird of paradise on the other side.

Cardio Interval—Plyo Power, Mountain Climbers

Time to work the abs and glutes again with cardio to melt away any fat over the muscle. Start by standing up. Do a right front kick leading with the knee, then exploding that powerful kick with the foot flexed, hands in ready fight position in fists by your chin. As you lower the leg, lunge back with the left foot. Support yourself by keeping your right hand on the right quad as you lower down to touch the floor with your left hand.

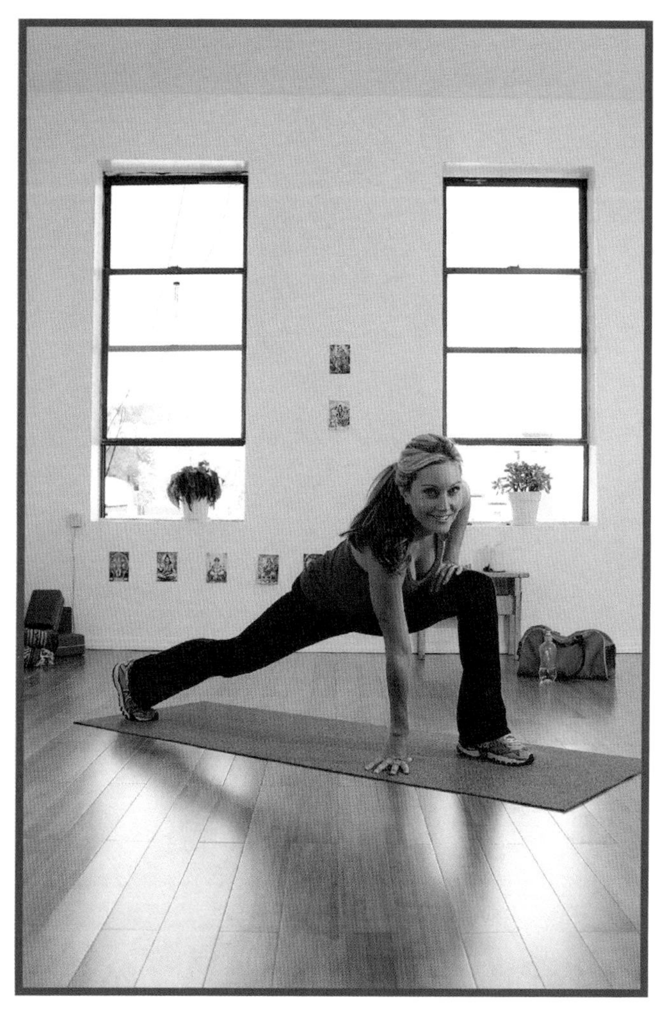

Trainer's Tip: Lunge far back so that your right knee is directly over the ankle as you reach for the floor.

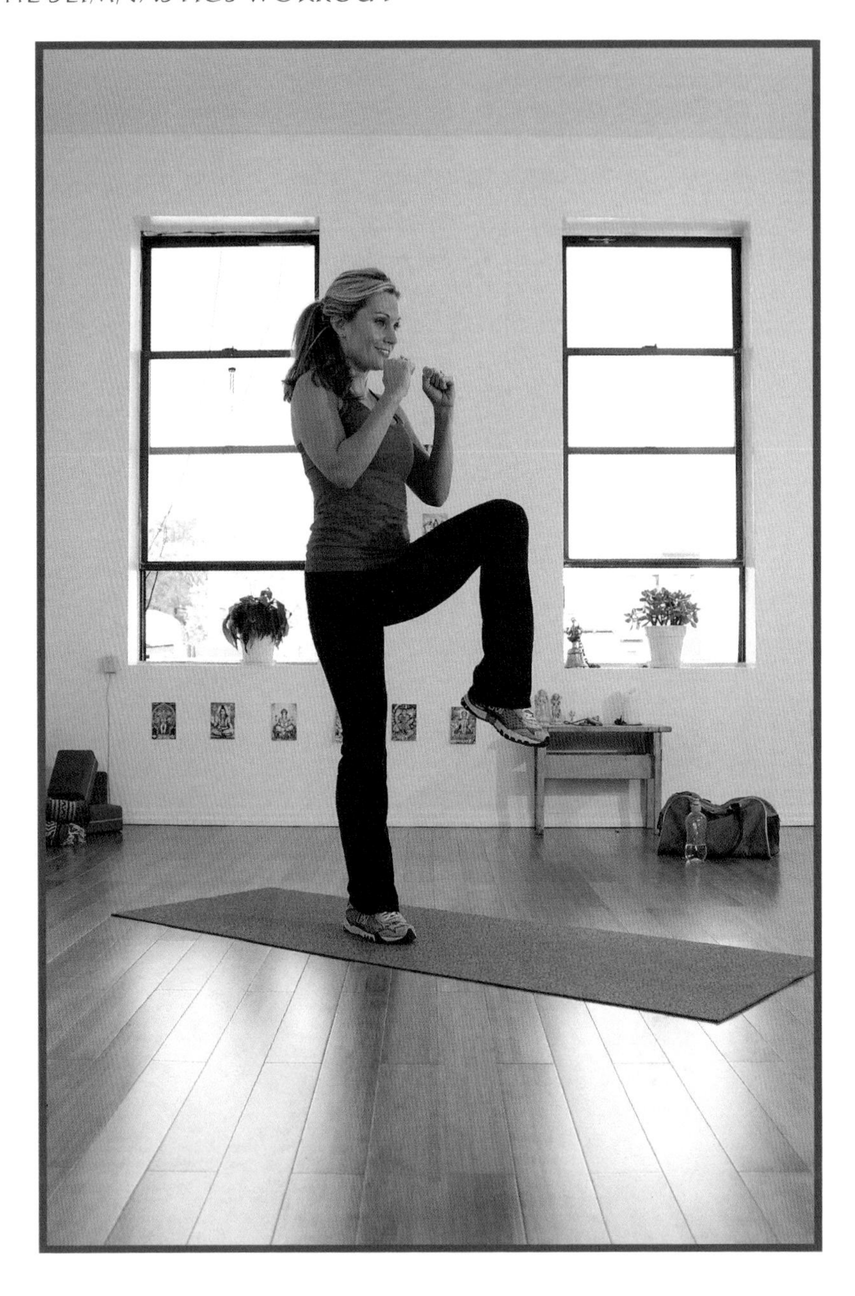

Hop back up for the second right kick by using your powerful leg and glute muscles!

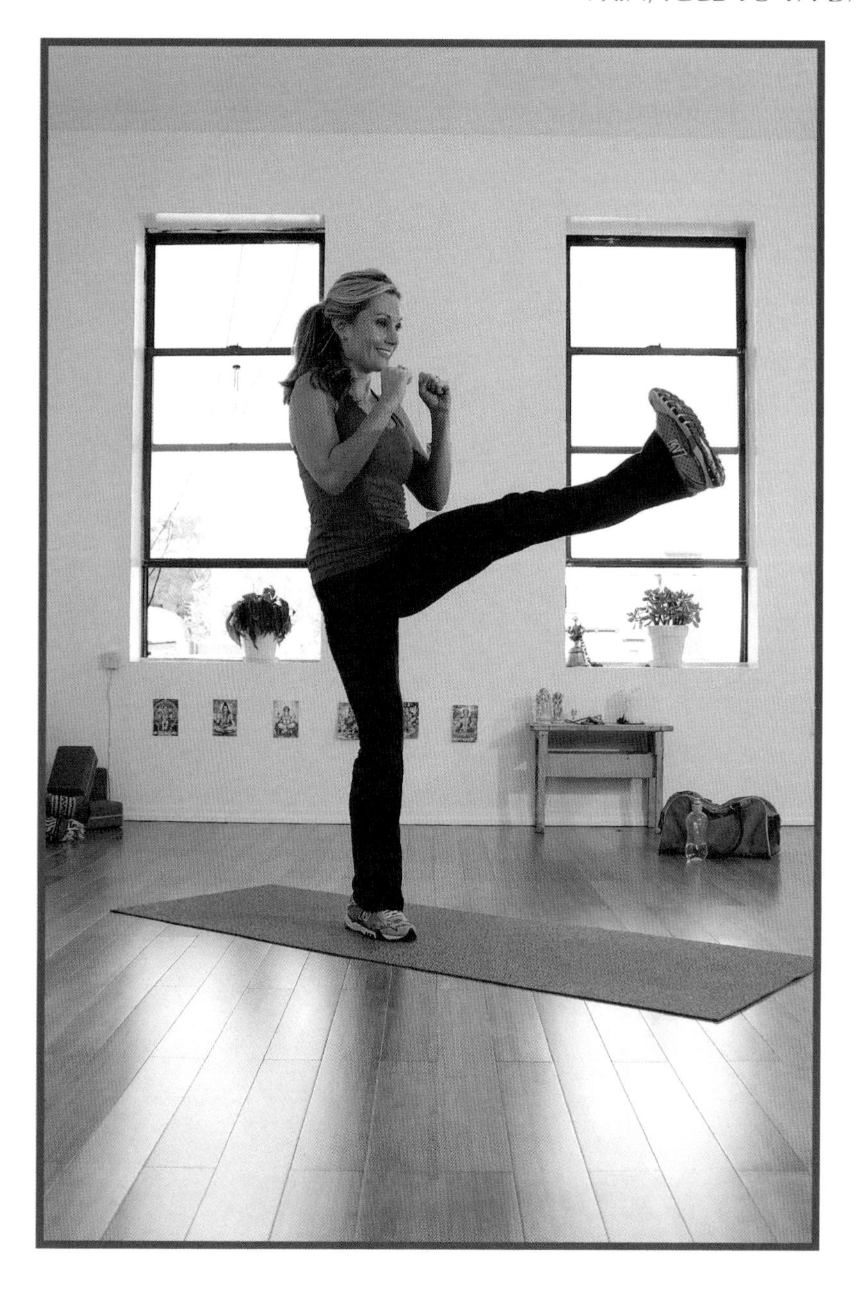

Do twenty on the right, twenty jumping jacks, then twenty on the left.

Mountain Climbers

To work the abs and continue the cardio burn, jump lightly onto the floor on your hands and feet into plank position.

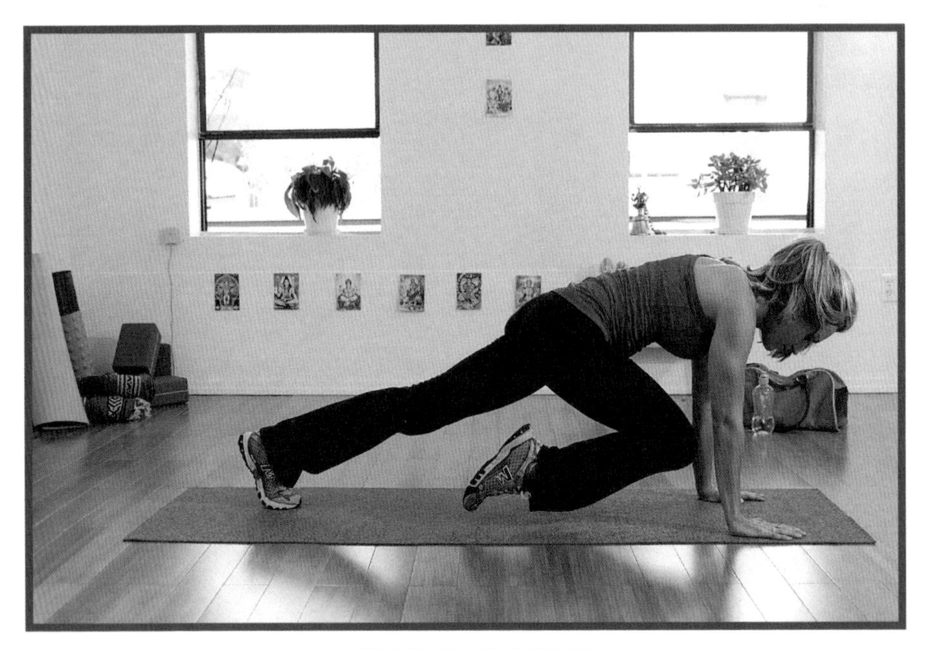

MOUNTAIN CLIMBERS

Keeping your gaze above your fingers and your hands directly under your shoulders, start "running" your knees in toward the chest one at a time, "climbing" the floor.

Recover with eight or more sunflowers.

Chapter 7

Detox and Diesel Arms and Legs

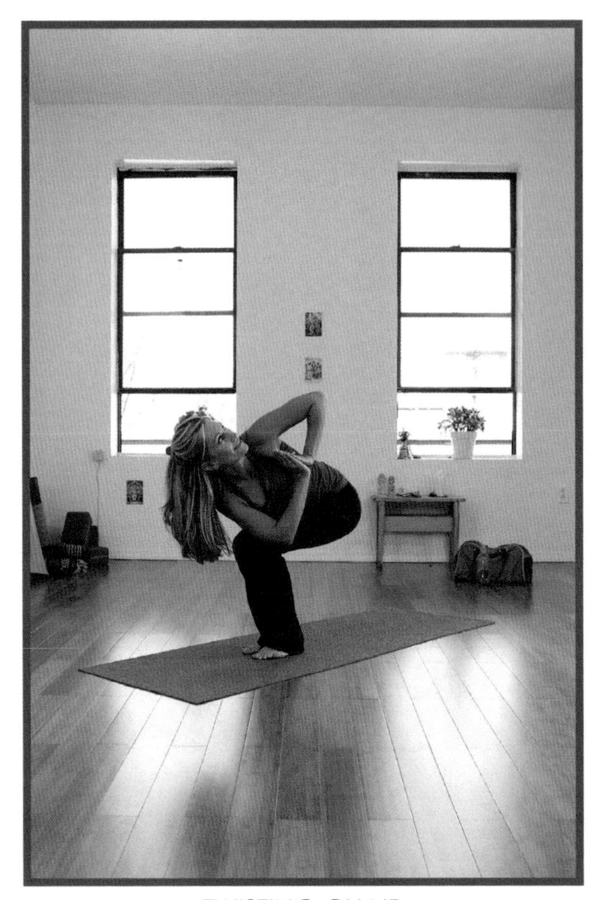

TWISTING CHAIR

Twisting Chair

This detoxifying twist is not only good for digestion and cleansing out toxins, it also tones leg and glute muscles as well. Start in standing mountain pose. With hands in prayer position, reach the hands to the sky and then sweep them down the center of the body and off to the right as you squat with both feet together into an imaginary chair behind you. Push your left elbow and triceps muscle into your right upper knee and quad and press your right hand into the left in prayer to deepen the twist. Look up to the sky over your right shoulder and contract your abs up and into your spine. Hold for three breaths and return to stand, sweeping hands overhead on the inhale and exhaling into the pose on the left.

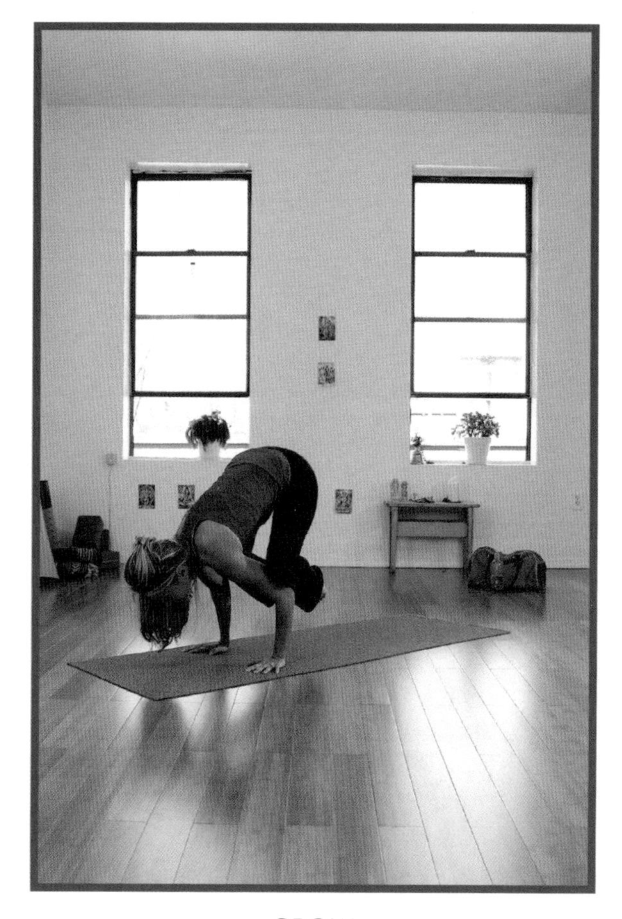

CROW

Crow

From standing in mountain after your twisting chairs, move to crow for upper body strengthening and balance. Start with feet hip distance apart and squat down, bringing the backside almost to the floor. Place your triceps inside the legs and your hands on the floor in front of you. Leaning forward onto the hands, lift hips high. Your arms become shelves for your shins and your legs hug your triceps. It is important to bend the elbows and gaze past your fingertips to the floor. Keeping your gaze forward will balance your center of gravity and avoid the tendency to fall forward. The toes lift off the floor towards one another. Hold for three breaths and come back down to your feet.

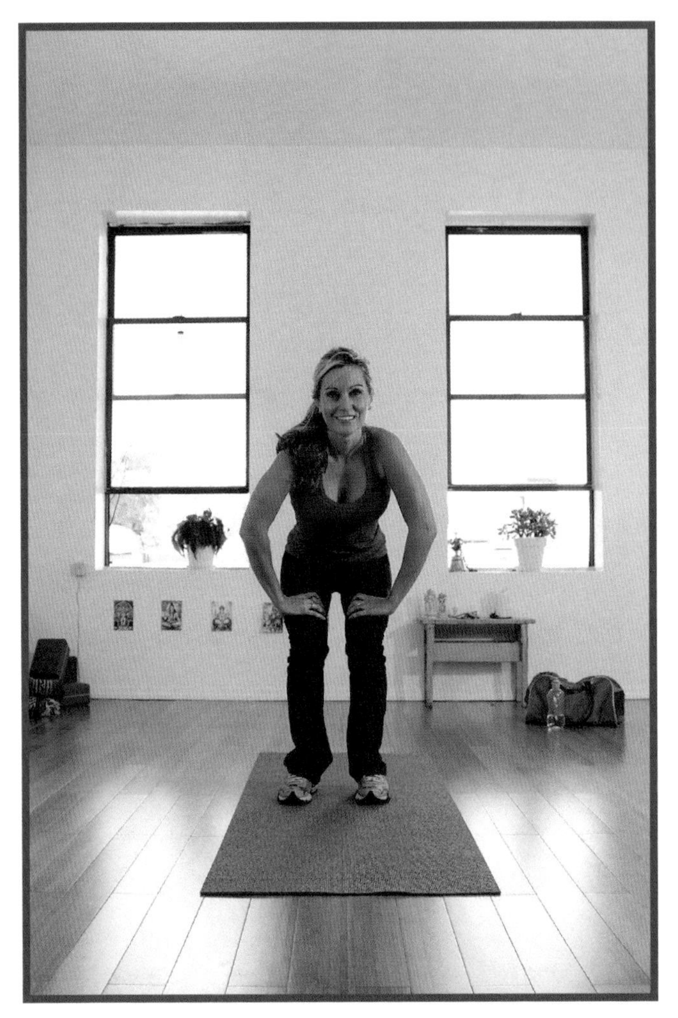

SPRING SQUAT PREP

Interval—Spring Squats

Between sides of the kick, put the feet closer together in shoulder-width squat prep. This time your knees will face forward. Place your hands on your quads with fingertips facing in and thumbs facing out.

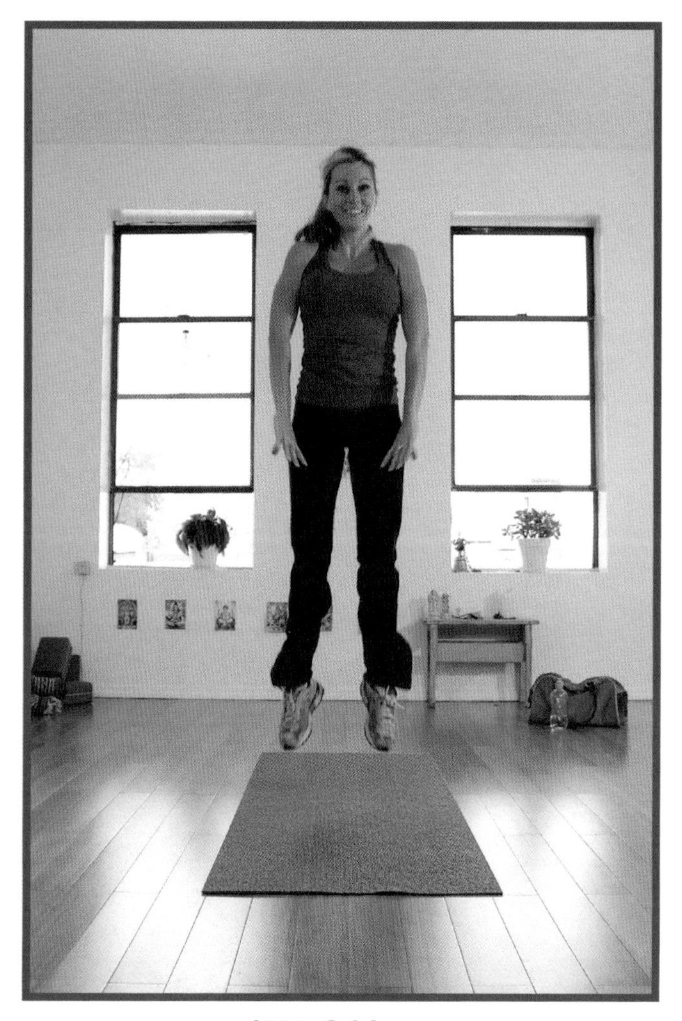

SPRING SQUAT

Squat low as if sitting into a chair and then "spring" off the ground by straightening the legs and using your muscle strength and plyometric power to leave the ground completely. Land softly, squatting into an imaginary chair, keeping hands on legs for support. Push off with legs again. Repeat ten times. Recover.

Chapter 8

Toning Twists

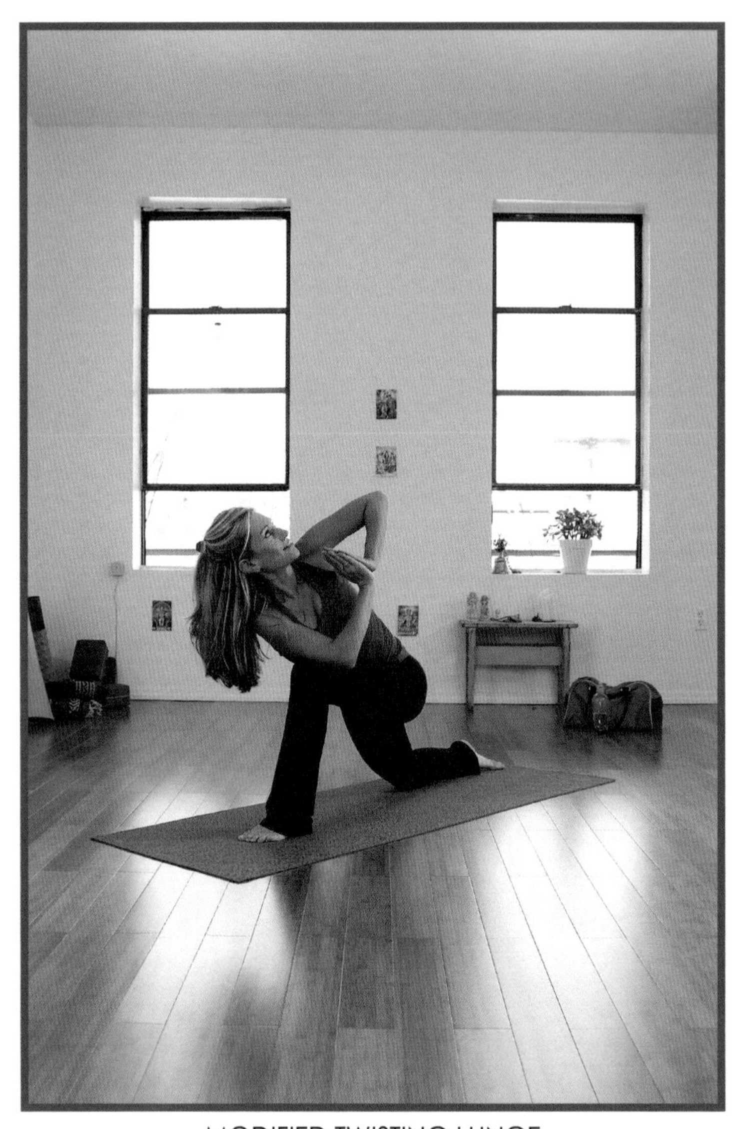

MODIFIED TWISTING LUNGE

Twisting Lunge

Stepping the right foot back into a lunge position with the heel off the earth, we sweep the hands off the floor and up into crescent lunge. The hands meet in prayer and then sweep towards the left knee and quadriceps.

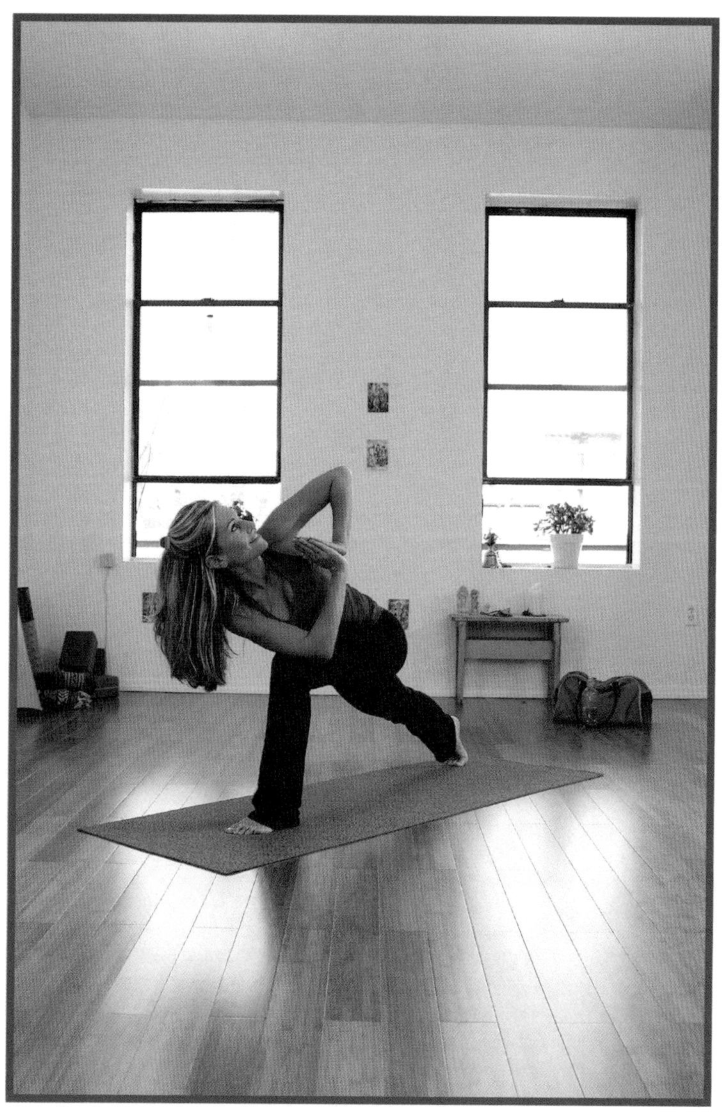

TWISTING LUNGE

As in chair, the triceps and elbow press into the leg and the palms press together allowing the abs to contract and the torso to twist and open to the left while gazing towards the sky.

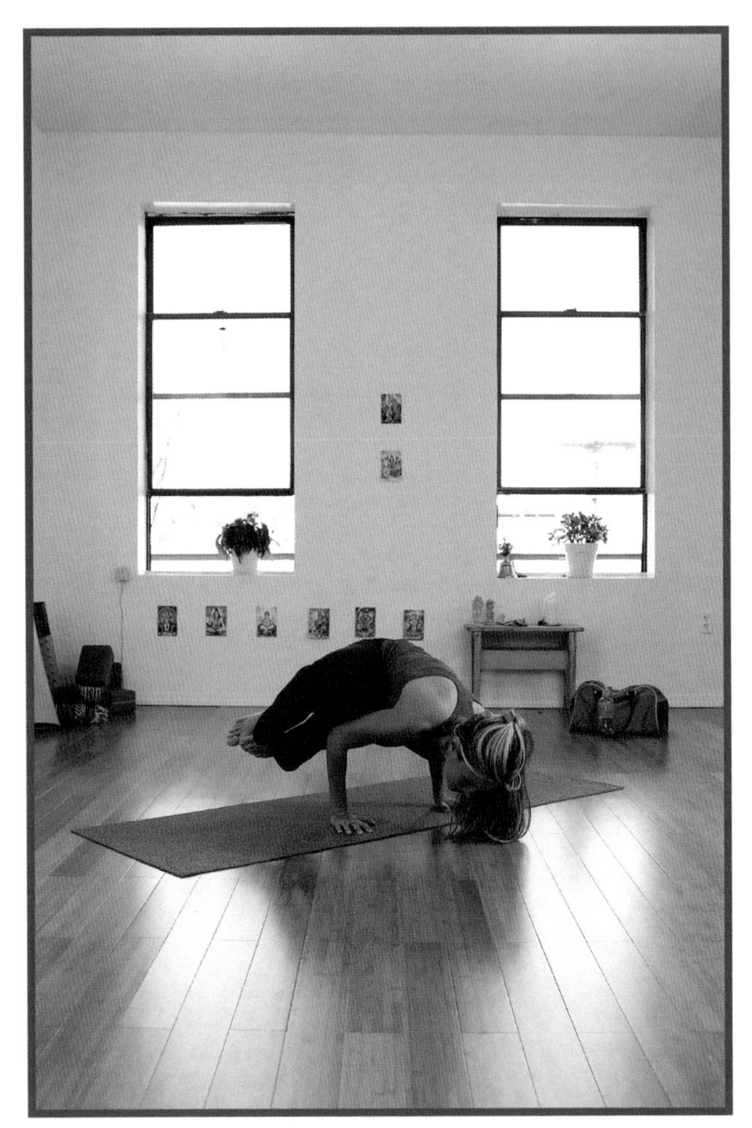

SIDE CROW PREP

Side Crow

Getting back into mountain with feet apart, prepare for crow as before, bringing the seat close to the ground, but this time place both hands off to the left side of the body, on the floor. Forming a shelf with your triceps again by bending the elbows, lean your body onto your arms and gaze onto the floor past the fingertips.

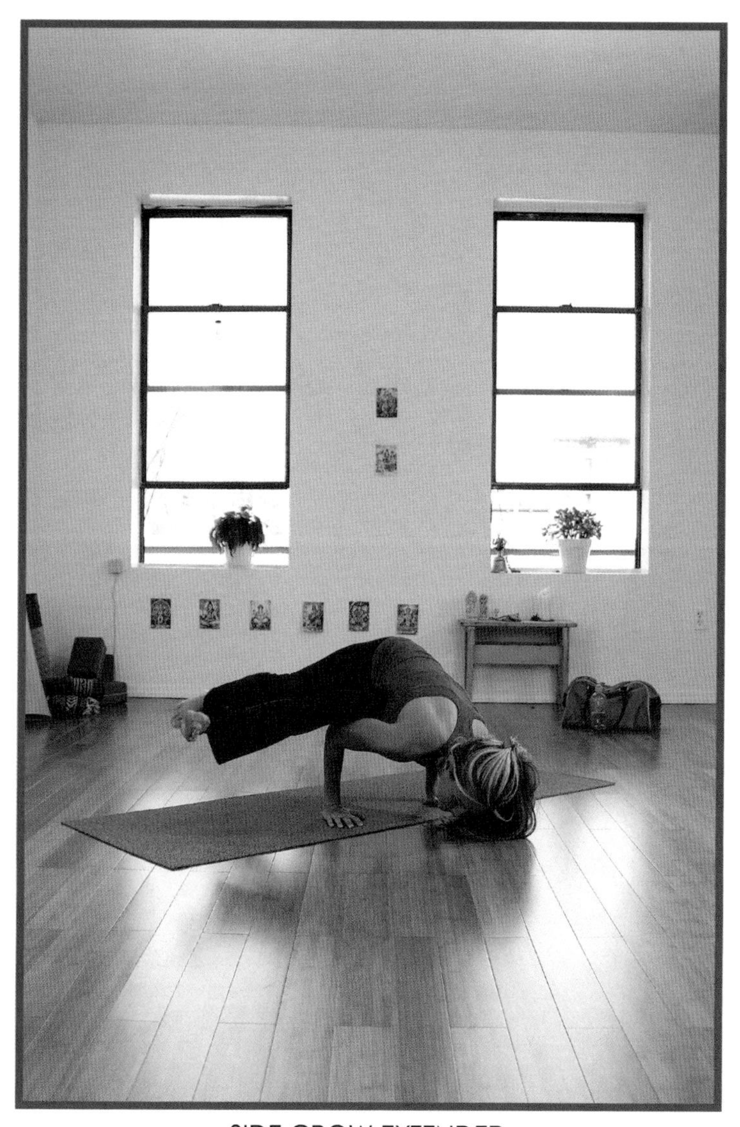

SIDE CROW EXTENDED

As the left thigh balances on the arms, the legs can slowly extend into side crow, out over the right side of the body towards the front of the mat.

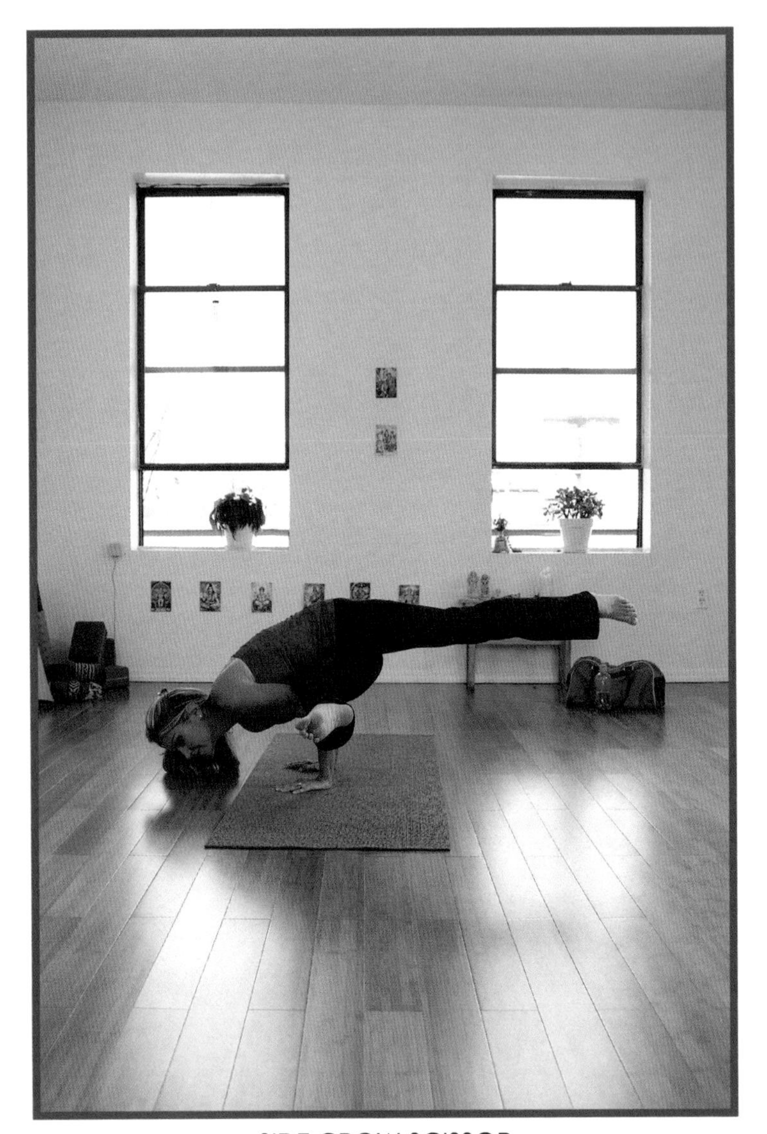

SIDE CROW SCISSOR

Another version allows you to extend your top right leg behind you while the left leg rests on the right tricep and reaches to the right of the body. Your legs will look like scissors, and the pose takes on a gymnastics quality.

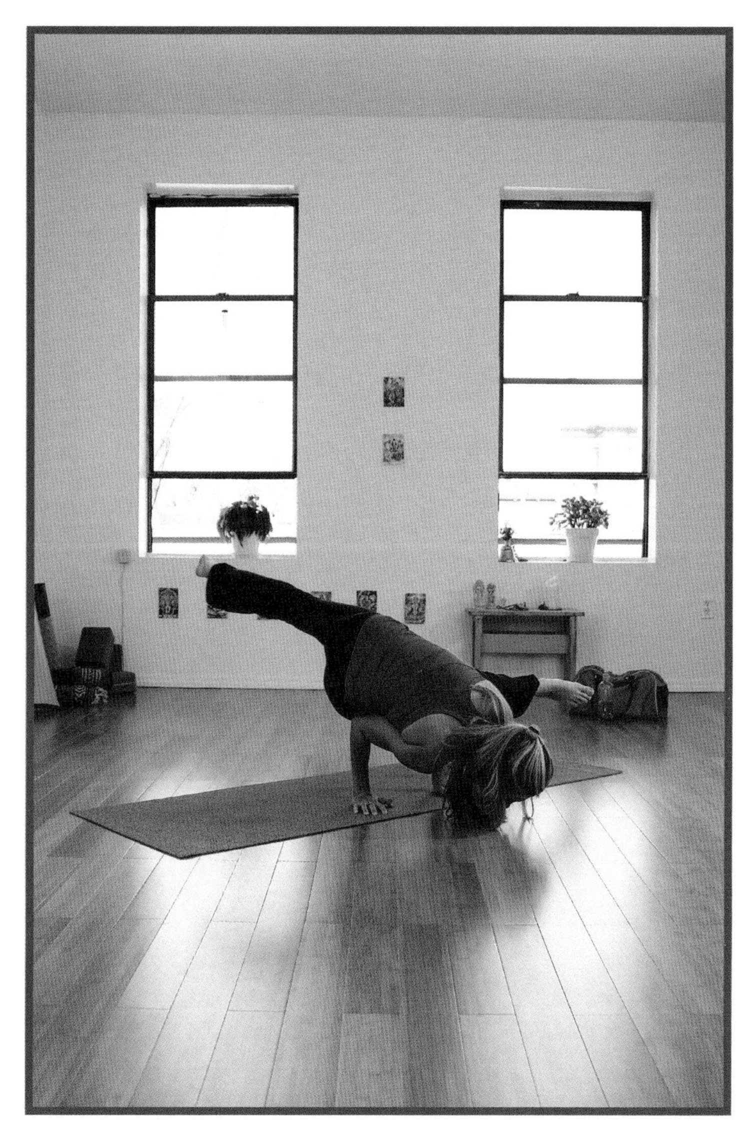

Hold for three breaths, release back to start, and repeat on the other side.

Cardio Interval—Side Kick Plie

Boost your booty with proper side-kick form!

Group fitness classes are most efficient when they can give you cardio and toning moves in one session, which is one of the reasons kickboxing remains so popular. However, the move that can provide the most bang for your booty-sculpting buck is the most common mistake made in cardio-kickboxing classes. Usually participants do a front kick to the side and call it a side-kick.

If done correctly, the side-kick will chisel your glutes and outer thighs; if done incorrectly, it just puts more stress on the hip flexor, a muscle that is already tight from sedentary modern life.

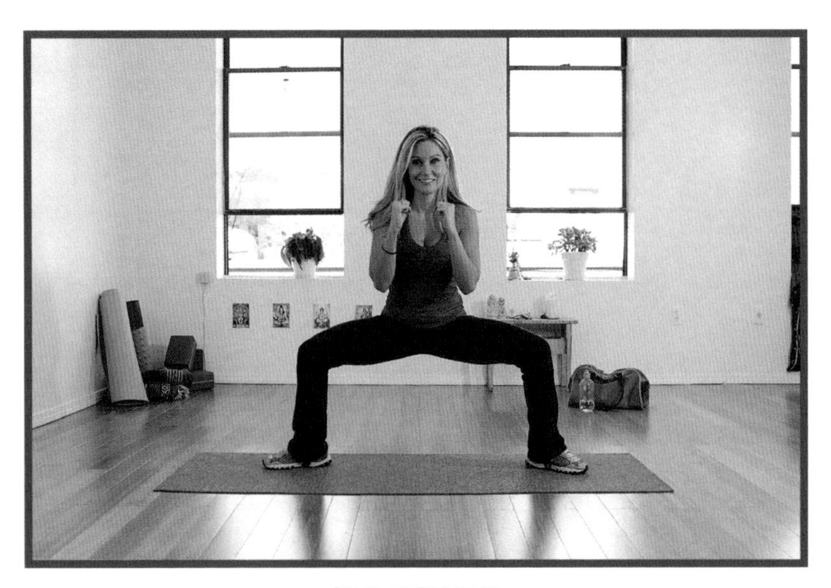

SIDE KICK PLIE

Stance: For a left side-kick, put your weight on your right leg with the knee and toe pointing out to the side at forty-five degrees.

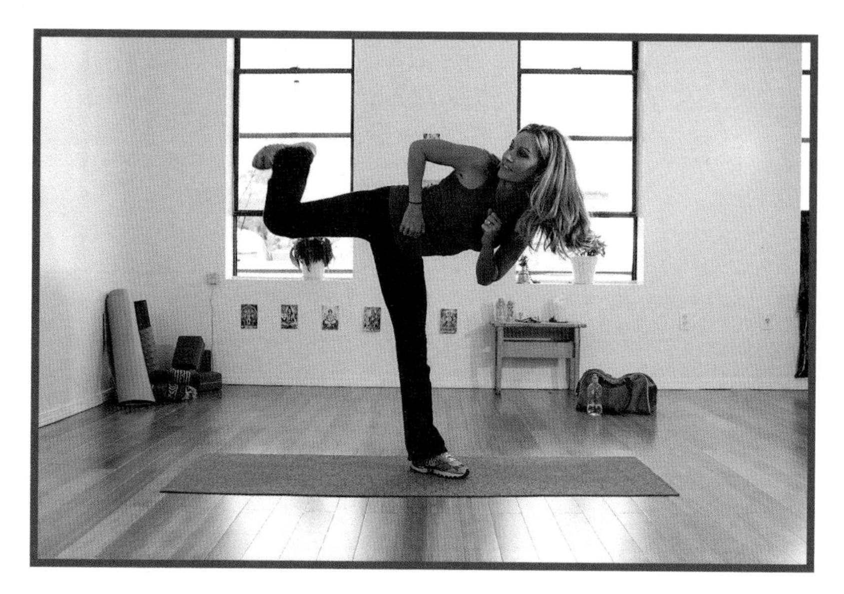

SIDE KICK CHAMBER

Chamber: Think of the kick in four counts. Count one is hinging at the hip and dropping your right shoulder to the right, kicking the core into action while bending your left leg and bringing the left knee toward your navel.

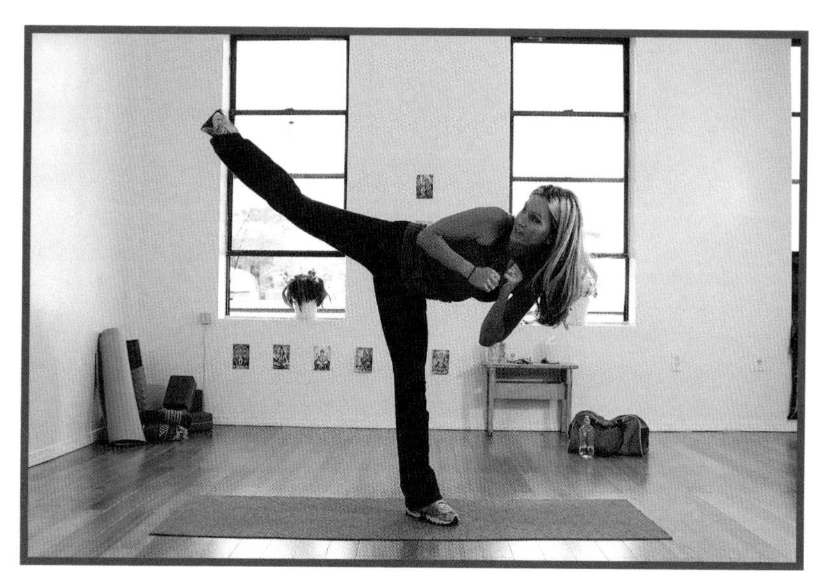

SIDE KICK

Impact: This is count two. The common mistake is for class participants to kick to the side with their toe pointing to the sky. To correct this, flex the foot and straighten the left leg and impact with your heel diagonally up and toe diagonally down. Think of it like this, if you're inside a room your heel should aim for the corner where the back wall and the ceiling meet. Your toe should point to where the floor and front wall meet on he other side of the room. Another way to visualize this is that your front hip bone or "front pocket" of your kicking leg should turn down towards the floor and your "back pocket" should be rotated up to the ceiling. Look at your foot with each kick to ensure appropriate form.

Retract: For count three, quickly retract the knee back towards the core and place foot back to the floor for count four.

Trainer's Tip: Adjust your target height. If you find it difficult to align your kick properly, instead of aiming for your opponent's head, aim for the stomach or knee. Master the foot alignment first, then work on the height. Even with a kick aimed at the (imaginary) opponent's knee, you are challenging your core and backside.

You've just mastered the booty-kicking side-kick.

Chapter 9

Legs off the Ground!

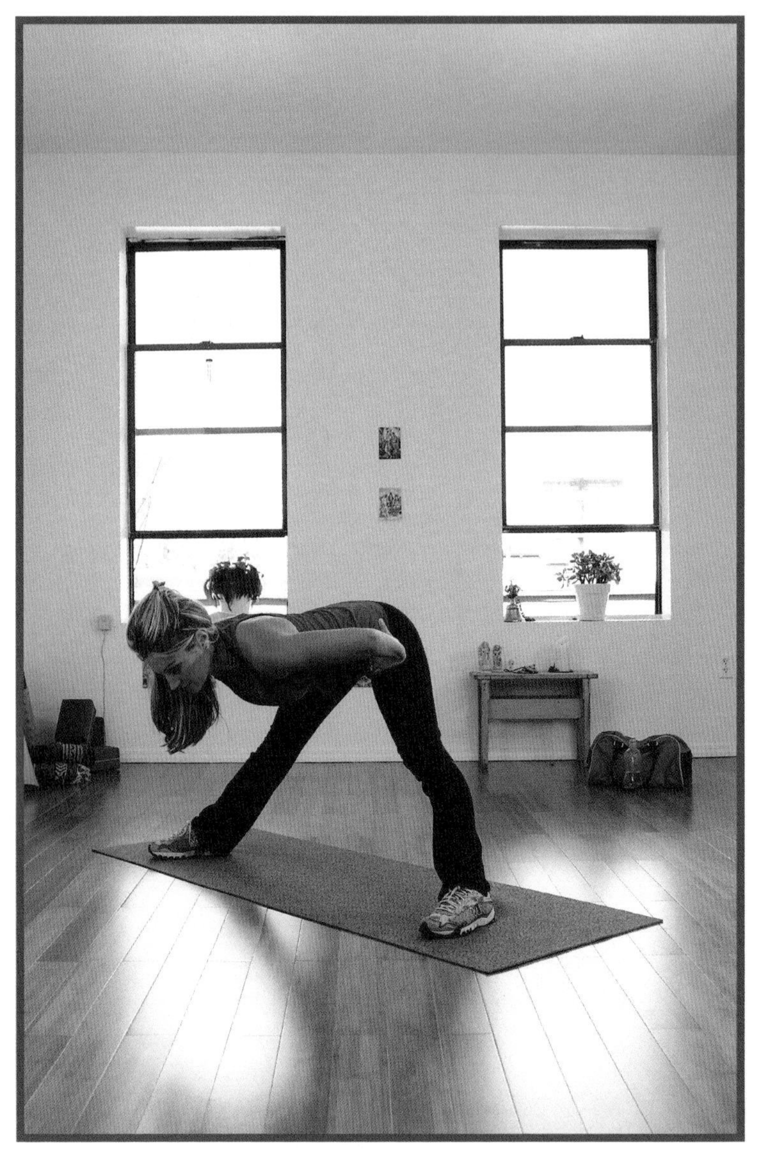

FIREFLY PREP STRADLE

Firefly:

This is another "ta-da" pose that builds strong arms, quads, and hip flexors as well as increases leg flexibility. Start in standing straddle, facing the long edge of the mat and widening legs more than shoulder width, about the length of one of your legs.

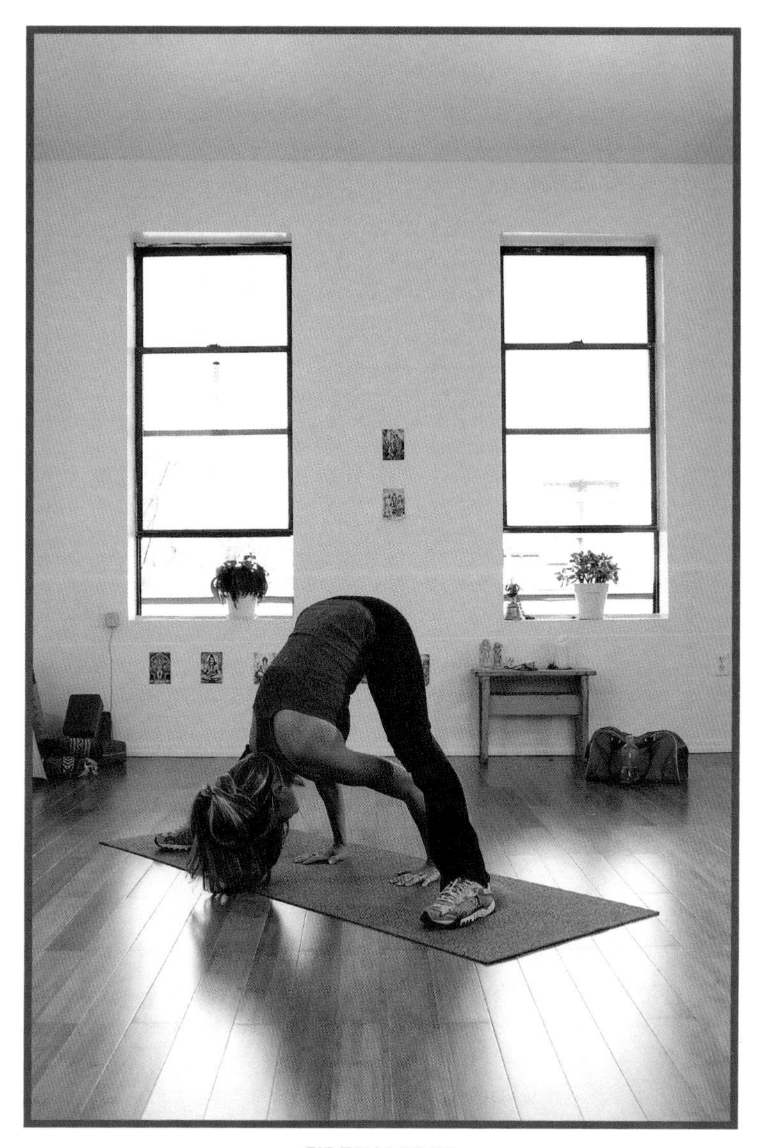

FIREFLY PREP

Hinging at the hips, you'll lower the torso towards the floor. Placing hands on the mat, hold the stretch for the hamstrings and inner thighs. If you can go deeper, you can choose to bend the elbows or move into firefly. Keeping the fingers pointing forward, walk the hands back underneath the body towards the back of the mat and bend the knees to "sit" above your elbows.

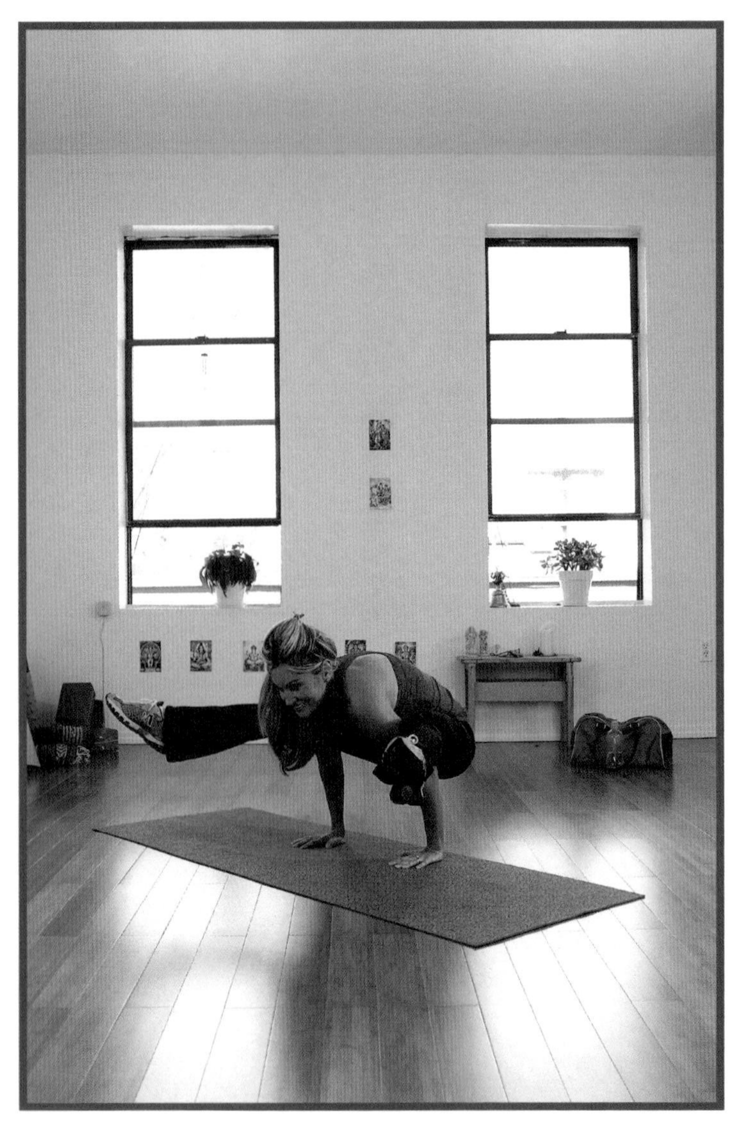

FIREFLY

Next, engage the front of the legs to lift the feet of the earth into *titibasana* or "firefly."

Dancer

Visual balancing poses bring the heart rate down and the mind in focus to prepare for soon-to-come upper-body burn and core-cutting to sculpt the arms without using weights, boost the bosom, strengthen the back, stretch the muscles, and shred the abdominals.

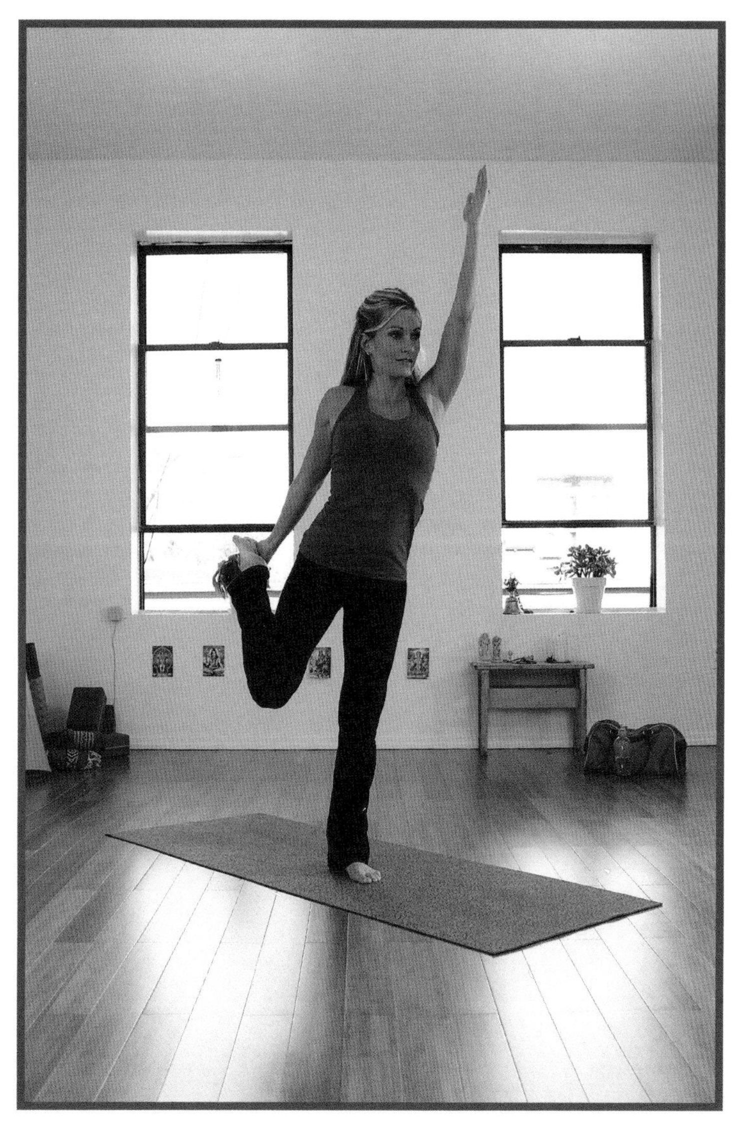

DANCER PREP

Begin in mountain pose and prepare to transform your body and mind into a free spirit of the dancer. Leaving behind expectations of how completely you've done this pose in the past, free the mind to go for it. Balancing on the right leg, bend the left knee and open your left hand so the palm is facing away from you. Wrap your fingers around your shoelaces and hold the quadriceps stretch for a breath or two.

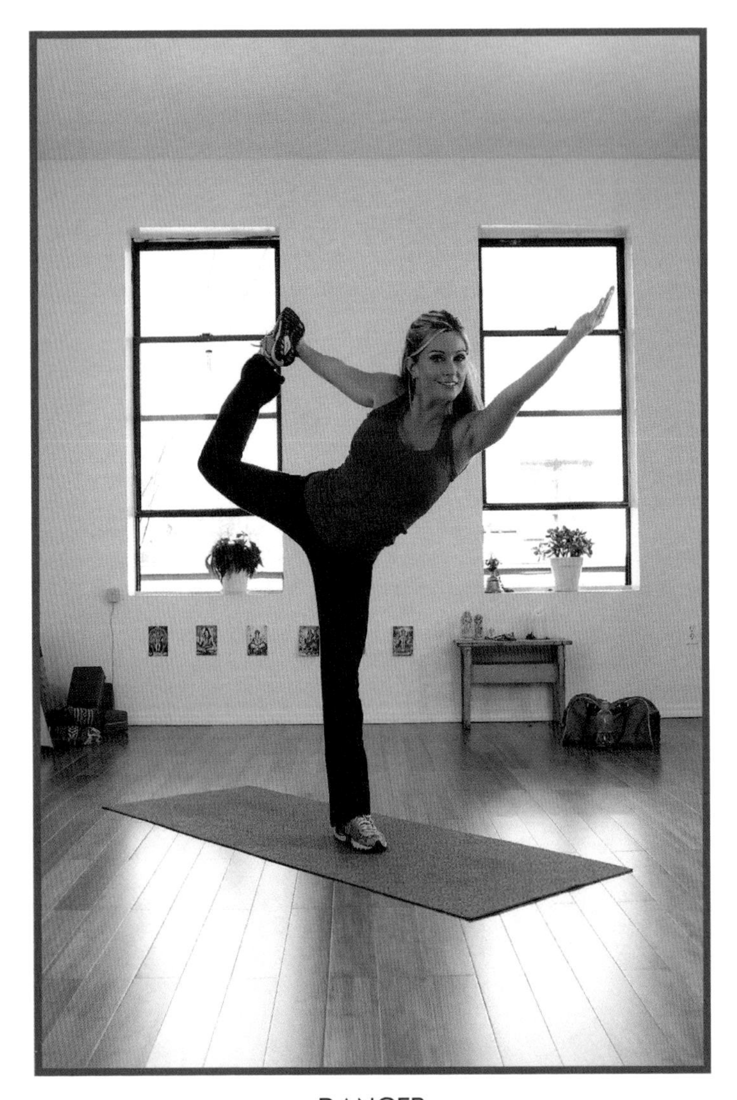

DANCER

Next, reaching the right arm to the sky, allow the left foot to push into the left hand as it straightens away and behind you. Your body will naturally tip forward a bit as your hand presses into the foot and the foot presses into the hand. (If you were facing a mirror, you might see your back toes peaking above your head, like a feather in your cap for attempting this fun backbend and ankle-strengthening stretch. Hold for three breaths, keeping the core tight and finding a focal point to stare at to assist in balancing. Return to standing and repeat on the other side.

Heel Stretch

In yoga we do a similar move with a "yogi toe lock," but here we do my favorite cheerleading style. Just think, it's easier on the ground than eight feet up balancing on a guy's wobbly hands! Stay grounded and stand tall!

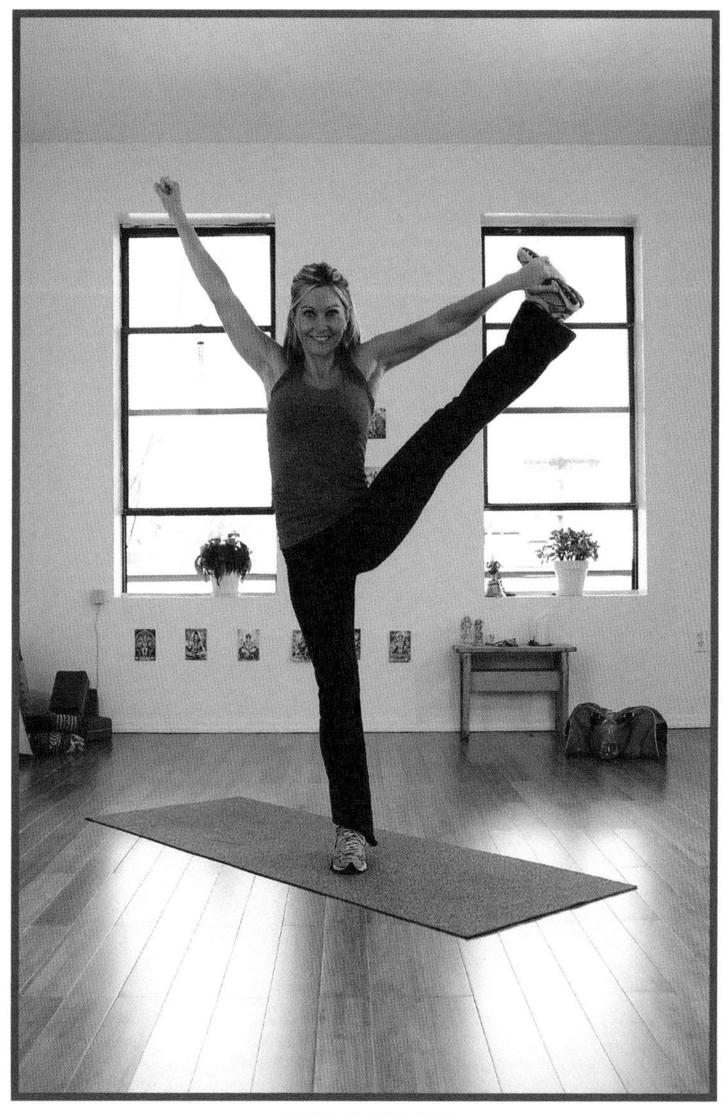

HEEL STRETCH

Begin by balancing again on the right leg and lift the left foot up towards the right inner thigh. Hold here to balance, then reach the left hand around the foot and push the leg forward, extending at the knee and working towards standing upright. Continue to breathe and open the leg towards the side while lifting it towards the sky. Breathe strength and stability into the standing leg and focus on the flexibility your left leg is gaining. Return slowly to standing after three breaths and repeat on the other side.

Cardio Interval—Jumping Lunges

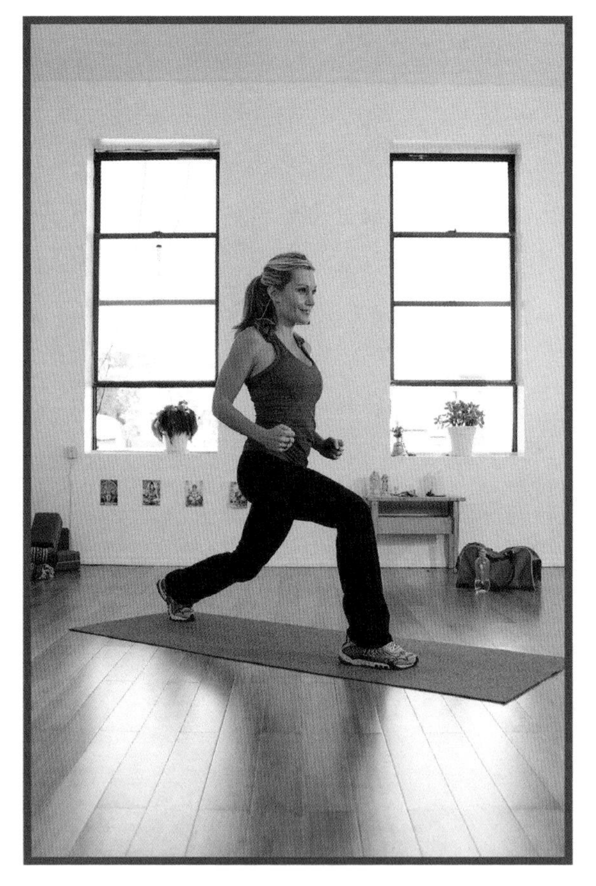

JUMPING LUNGE RIGHT

This simple move takes a right lunge, then you jump up in the air to scissor the legs and land with the left leg in front in a lunge.

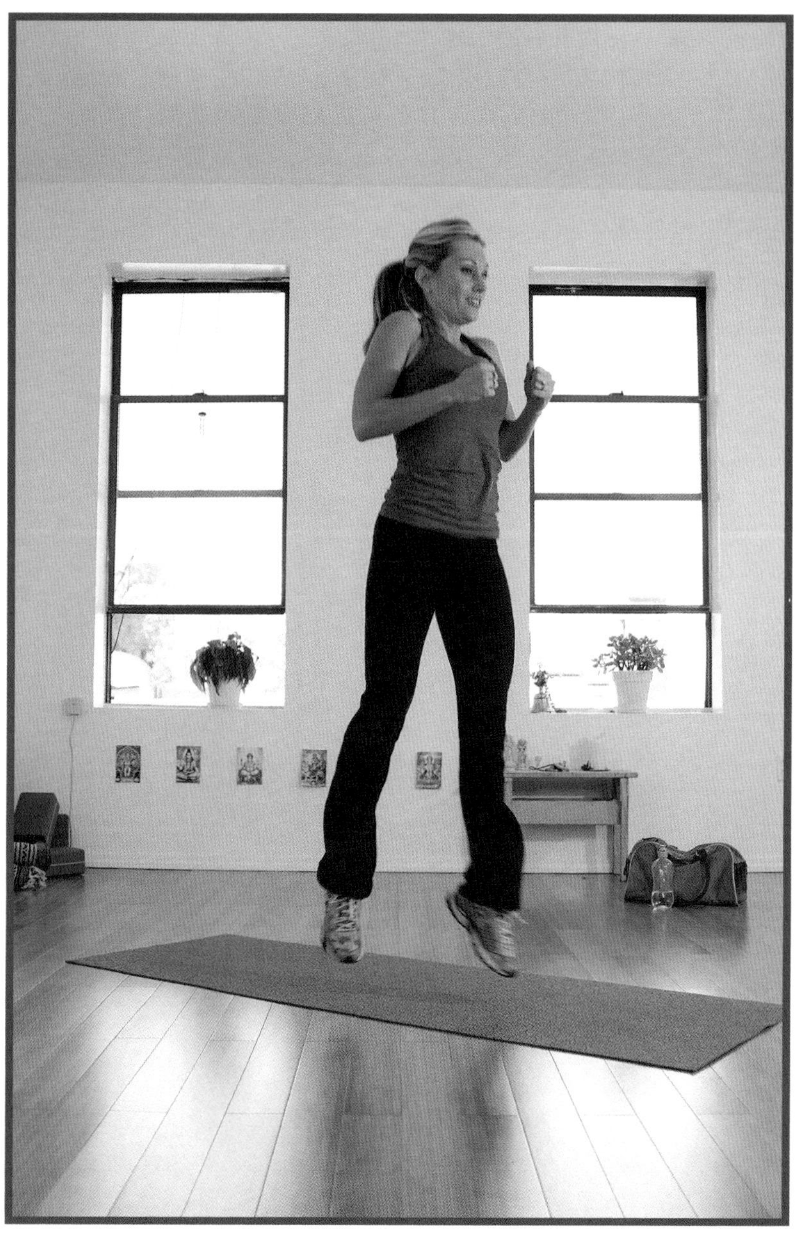

JUMPING LUNGE CHANGE

Do ten repetitions (landing right then left in front equals one).

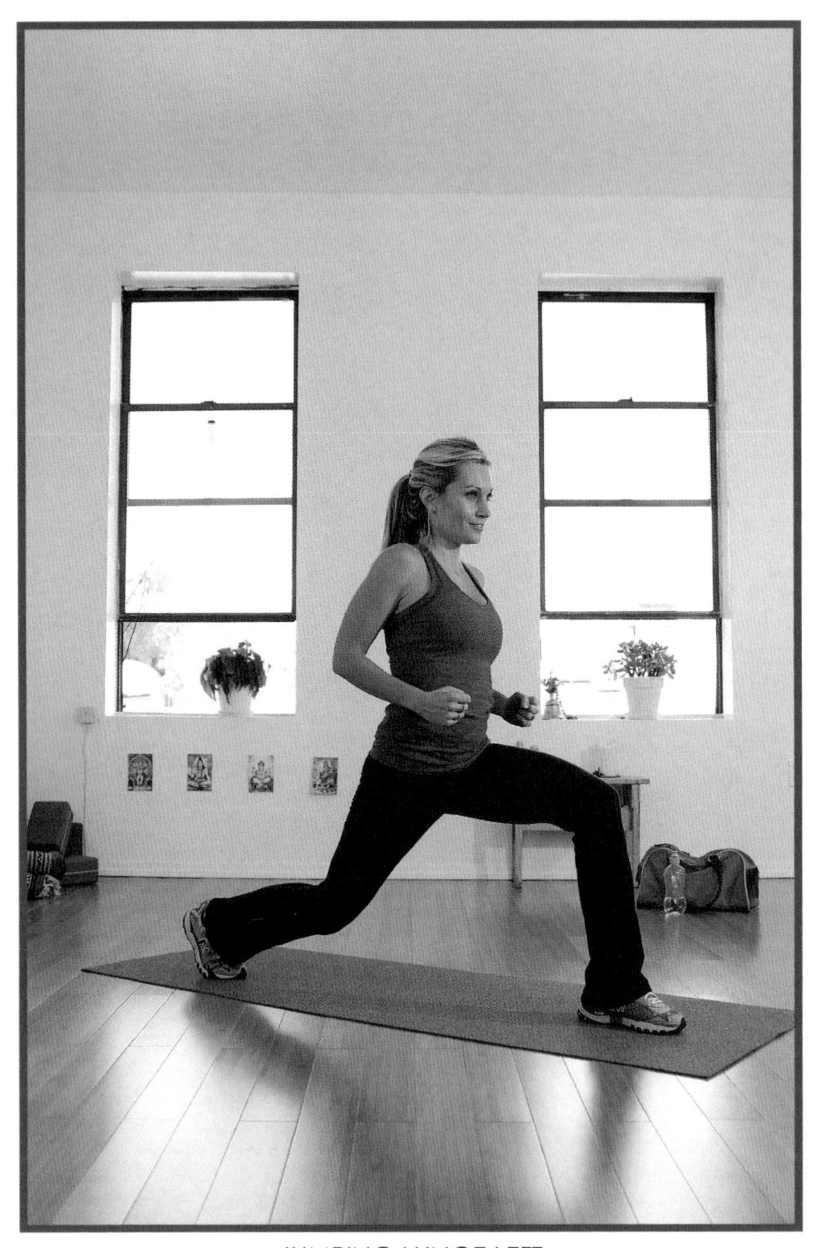

JUMPING LUNGE LEFT

Chapter 10

Balance and Butt Kicking

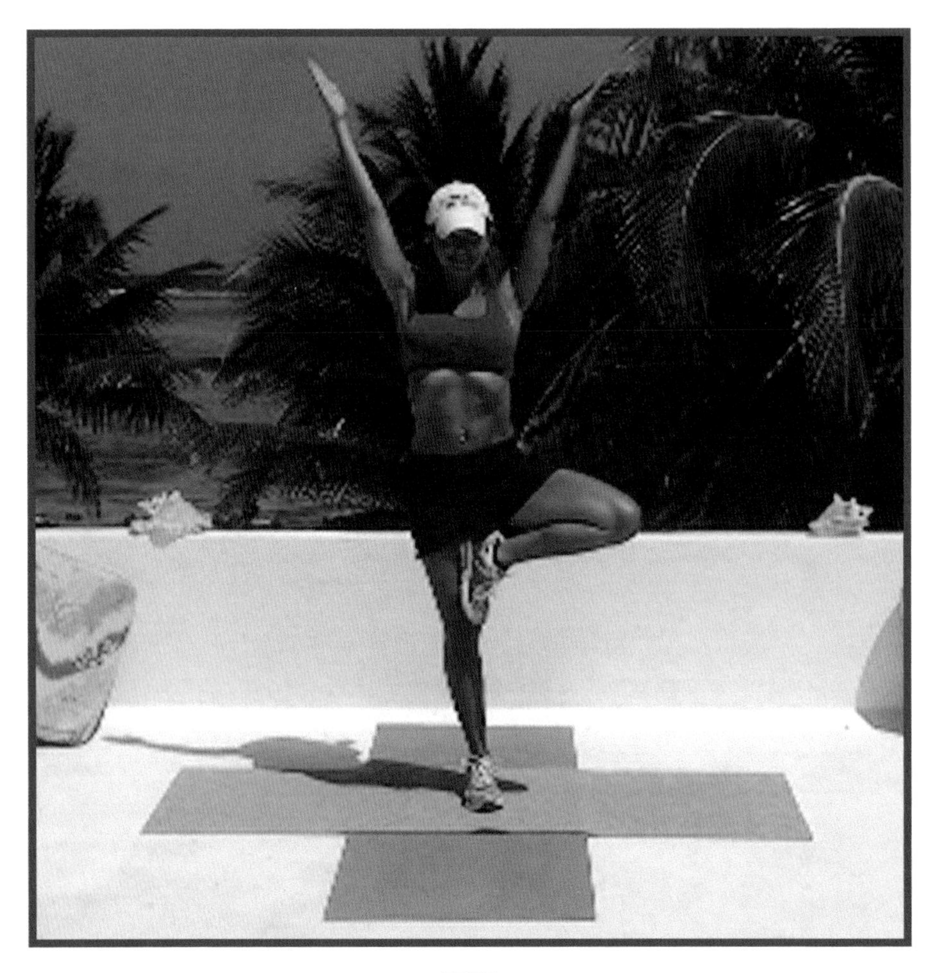

TREE

Tree

Balancing on the right leg, slowly lift the left foot to the inside of the right calf or right thigh, avoiding the knee.

By pushing the foot into the leg and the leg into the foot, you can find balance in the pose. Lift the hands into prayer at the heart, then over the head, opening the branches into a V if you choose. If your branches sway in the wind, remember it is normal—focus on a fixed point with your eyes, breathe, and root into the ground for balance. Hold for three breaths and move directly into warrior III pose without lowering the leg.

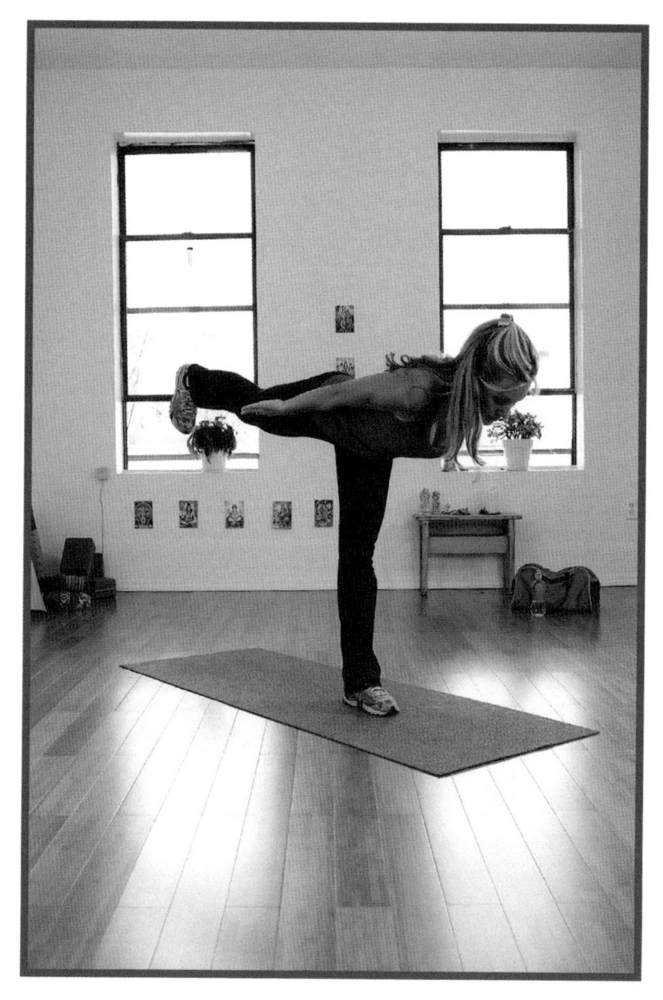

WARRIOR III

Warrior III to "Yoga Butt Plank Flow"

This is a great ankle and glute strengthener for yoga legs and booty.

From tree position, shift the left knee to the front and then slowly kick the foot behind you, hinging at the hips. Allow the torso to lower so that the extended back leg and shoulders are parallel with the earth. You may choose to extend the arms straight in front, to the sides, or next to the hips while shining a light through the crown of the head and keeping the spine in line.

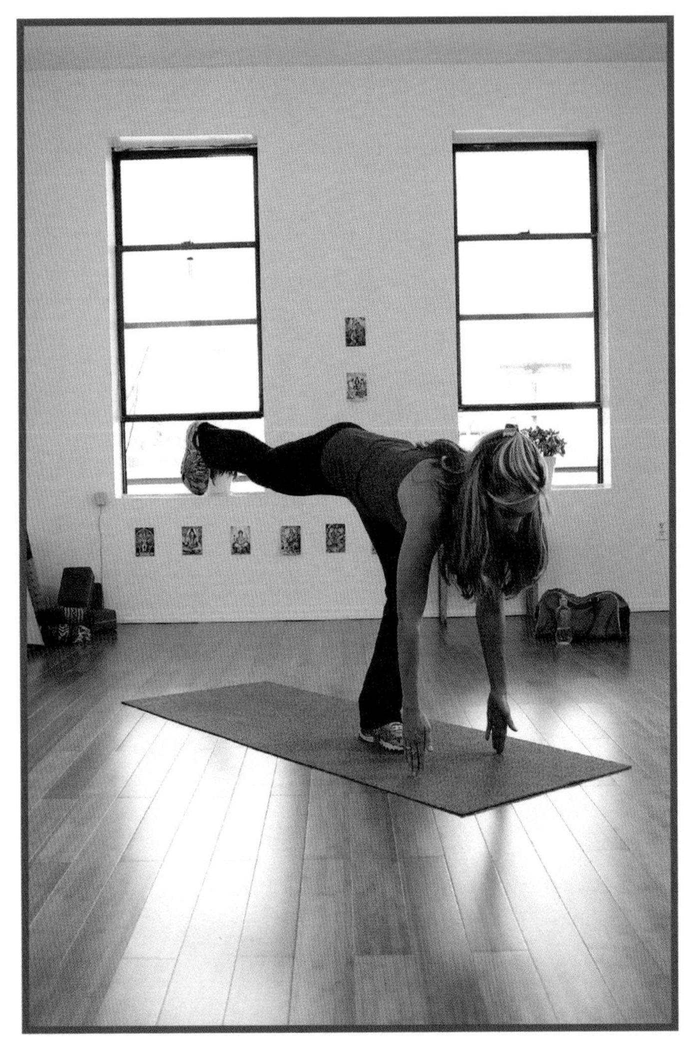

WARRIOR III BOOTY BOOST

Hold for three breaths and then lower the hands to frame the right foot while bending the right knee. Allow the left foot to anchor down onto the floor behind you and step the right leg back into plank position. Hold for one breath. On the next inhale, lift the hips and sweep the right leg back between the hands and rise back into warrior III with hands at heart center. Lower into plank five more times and then rise into mountain.

Repeat tree, warrior III, and "yoga butt plank flow" on the other side.

Cardio Interval—Jump Rope to High Knees/ Jump Tuck to Kick Butt

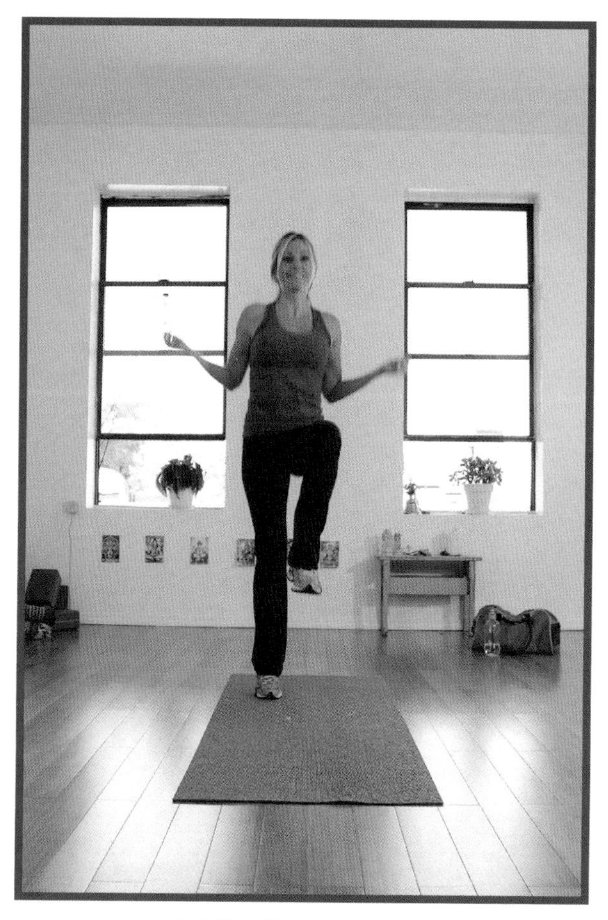

JUMP ROPE KNEES UP

Start by simulating a jump rope by twirling your hands and using the biceps to move your "rope" while kicking your heels up and behind toward your glutes. Repeat twenty times and then bring the knees up during the jump rope interval to the height of your belly button. You can even move your hands so the palms face the floor at belly button level with bent elbows and bring your knees to tap your hands. Repeat for twenty. Return to a "butt kick" jump rope move to recover for twenty counts.

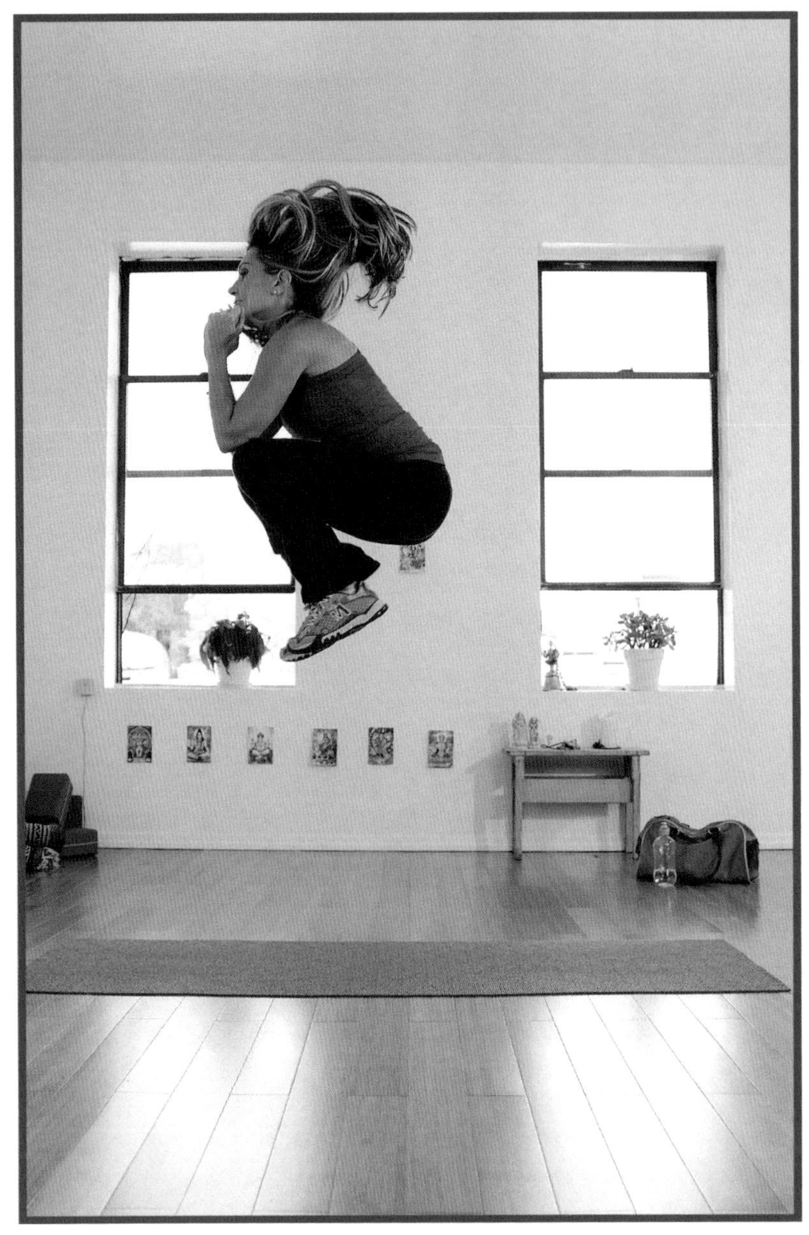

JUMP TUCK

Then jump both knees to the belly button in a jump tuck motion, as in cheerleading and gymnastic tucks.

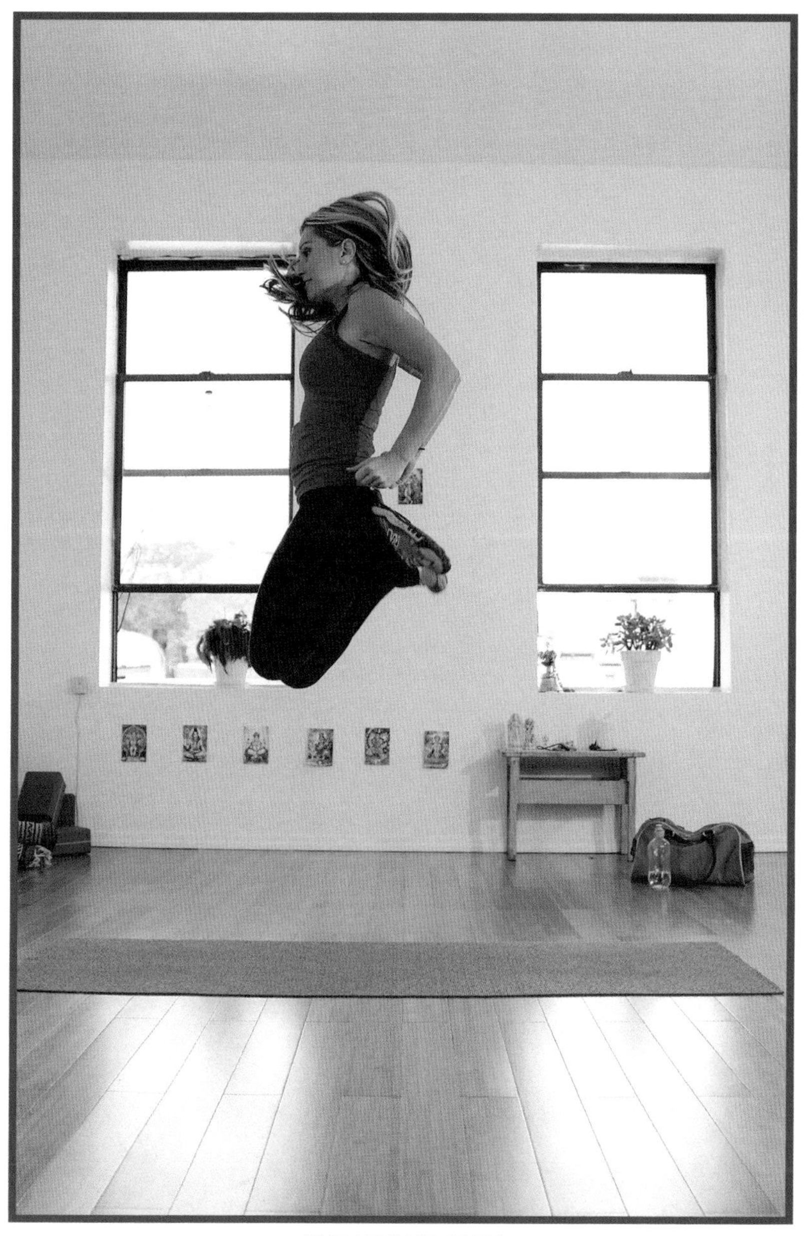

KICK YOUR BUTT

Do one tuck and one butt kick. Repeat ten times and then return to a jump rope motion to recover.

Cool down with sunflowers.

Chapter 11

Upper Back and Inner Thighs

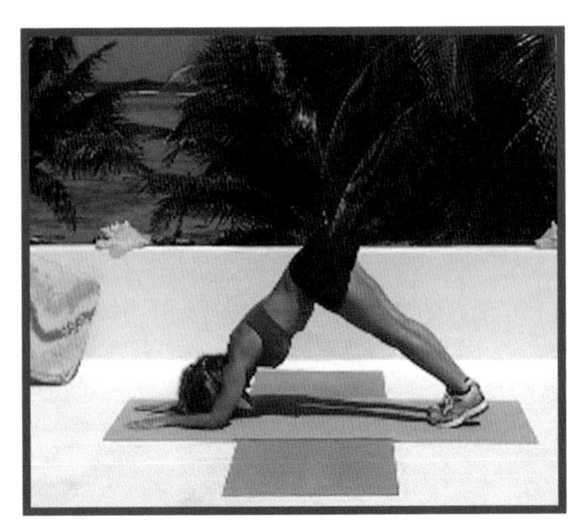

DOLPHIN

Swimming Dolphin

This move works your core, upper back, and shoulders while stretching the legs. Start on all fours and lower your elbows onto the floor. Lift the hips to the sky by straightening the knees.

Drop the head between the shoulders and look at your knees. Keeping the core engaged, move forward so that the shoulders move over the elbows and you are in a forearm plank position. Then use your upper back, core and shoulder strength to push back into an inverted V.

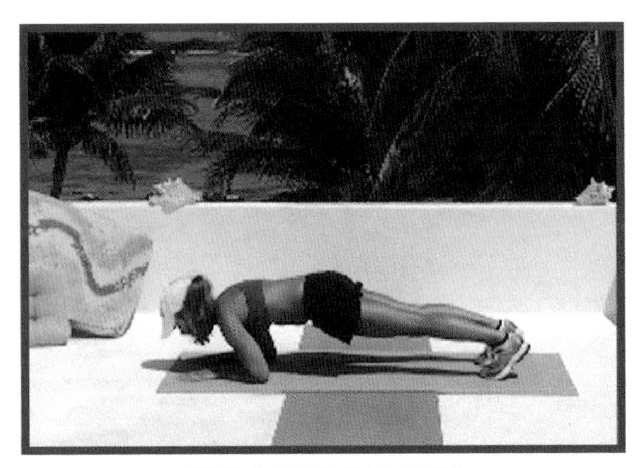

SWIMMING DOLPHIN

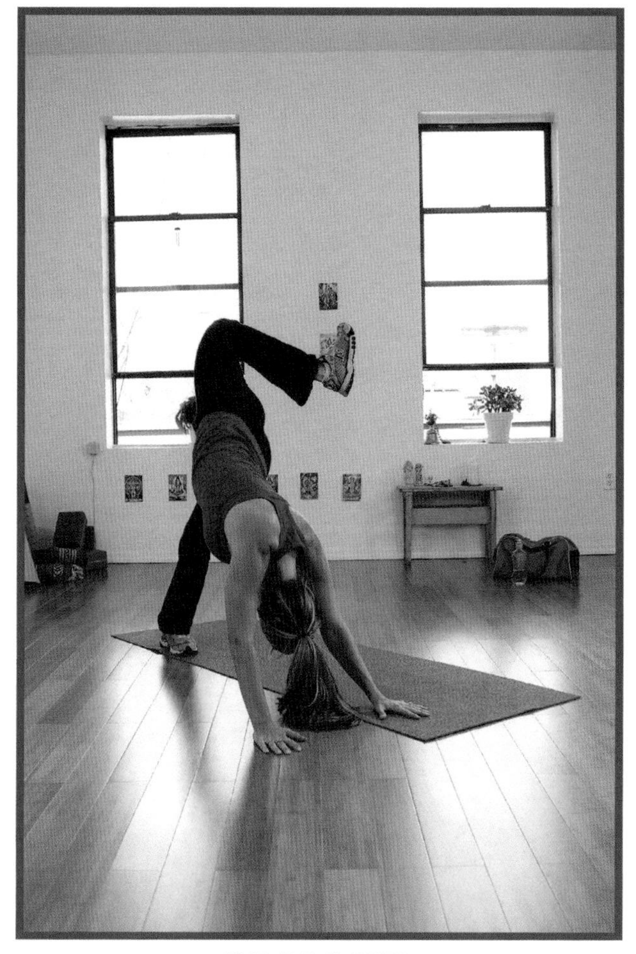

FLIP DOG PREP

Make It Harder: When moving hips back towards feet, lift off your elbows into a down dog and lift one leg. Swim forward into dolphin with one leg hovering off the floor, push back to down dog, and switch legs.

Rockstar

From down dog, lift the right leg off the floor and open the hip while bending the right knee, so that if you looked under your left armpit you might see your right heel. Shift the weight into the left hand and allow the right foot to continue backward and towards the floor while the right hand lifts of the floor.

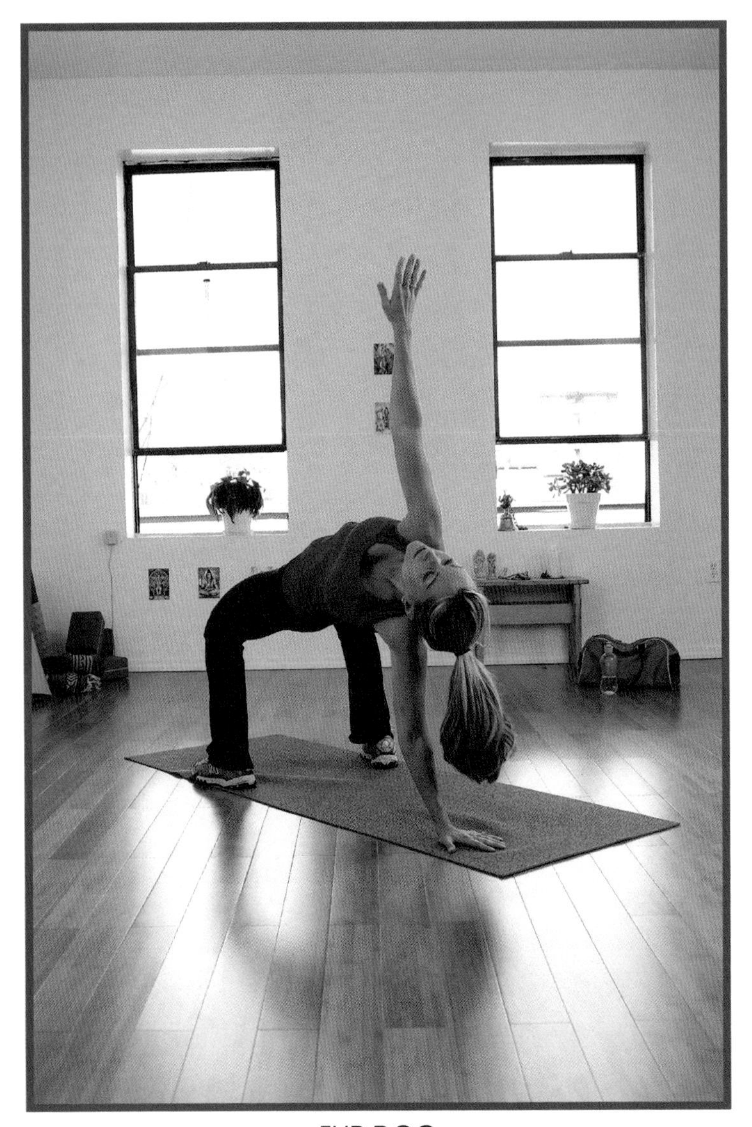

FLIP DOG

Land on the right foot into a three-legged wheel and look at your right hand outstretched and overhead. Quickly place the right hand onto the floor and flip the left fingers to face the shoes to complete your wheel as you transitioned from down dog to wheel like a rockstar!

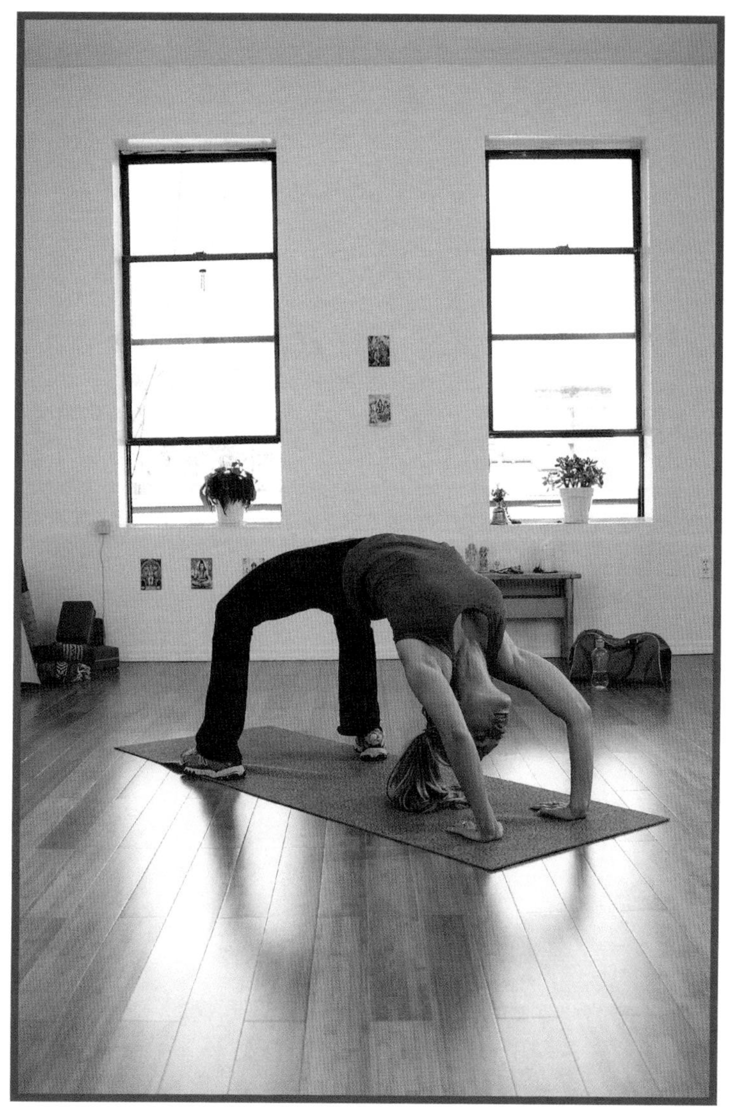

WHEEL

You may chose to rest on your back and hug the knees into the chest before repeating on the other side or flip that dog back over by lifting your right leg off the floor and pushing through your left arm, engaging the core to turn back over and land the right arm and leg back into down dog. (You can see the move in real time on my Slimnastics DVD, Amazon.com.)

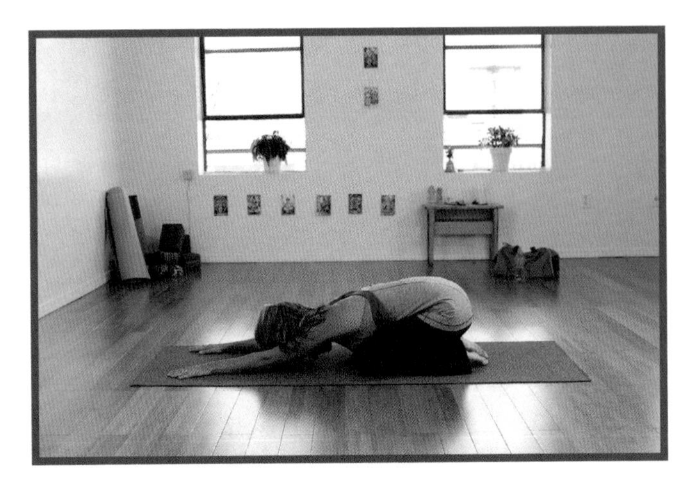

CHILDS POSE

Recover in **Child's Pose** or do wheel push-ups before flipping back over. Then repeat on the other side.

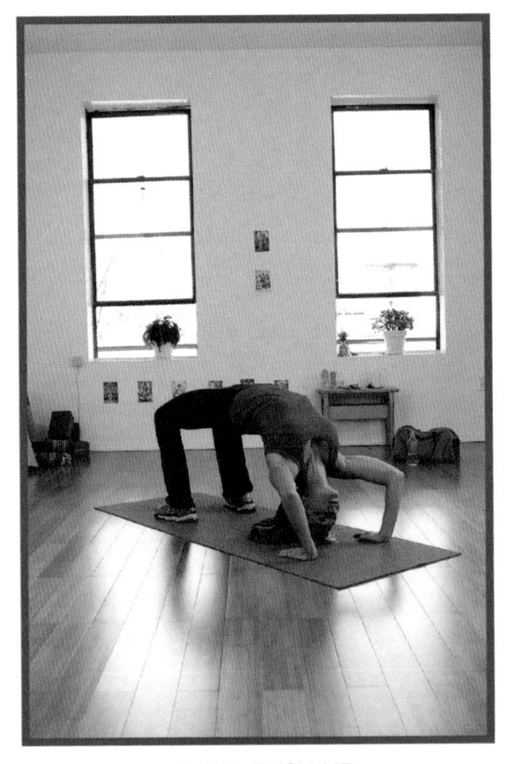

WHEEL PUSH UP

Wheel Push-ups

The wheel push-up is my favorite upper back move because it requires no equipment, and I always feel the muscles getting sore and stronger afterward.

Everyone knows about push-ups—their convenience and effectiveness—but what about the opposing muscle group?

Working your upper back, trapezius, and rhomboids usually requires machines, free weights, or tubing and a personal trainer forcing you to do them and with correct body alignment. Everyone from military men to desk job devotees to new moms tend to get the back slump that comes from either overdoing the push-ups without working the upper back, over-stretching the upper back at a computer or in the car in a slumping position, or holding a baby all day.

If you've done the regular wheel in yoga class, this will feel familiar. If you have never done a wheel, I will walk you through it.

Lie on the floor on your back, looking up at the sky. Bend your knees and place your feet on the ground. Flip your hands so that they are on the ground next to your ears with fingertips pointing to your feet. Try to lift yourself up with your arms gently onto the crown of your head. Hold there without putting pressure on the head or neck, and then slowly lower down and counter-stretch your back by hugging the knees to your chest for 10 seconds.

If you feel strong enough, perform the move again, and this time lift off the head and straighten the arms and legs as much as you can, as if someone tied a string around your waist and is pulling your belly to the sky. Hold this arch (the wheel) for 2 to 10 seconds and repeat the counter-stretch above.

If you are ready for the wheel push-up, go back through the first two progressions, and once in the wheel position with arms and legs straightening into the arch formation, start bending the elbows to just barely tap the head to the floor and then straighten the arms again. That is one push-up. Work up to doing fifteen at a time and always counter-stretch between sets.

Cardio Interval—Jacks to Plies/Plie Clap Feet

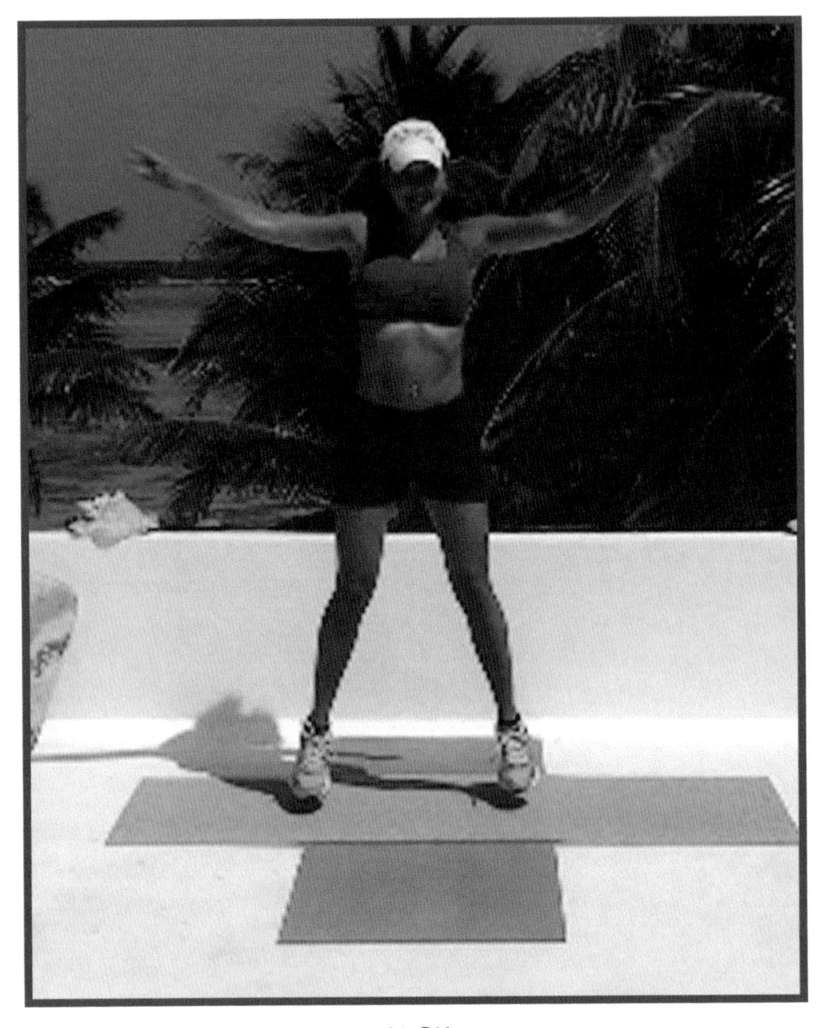

JACK

Perform ten jumping jacks, and then do a jack, bring the feet in and hands down, and land the feet out to the sides so that the toes point to the corners of the mat and the knees are directly over the ankles, quads parallel to the floor.

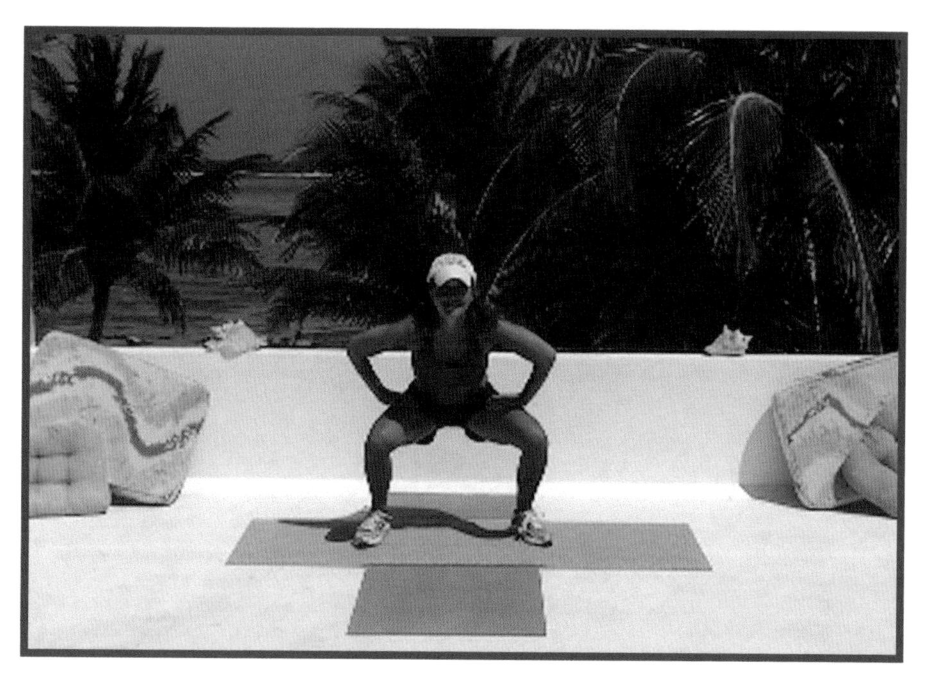

JACK PLIE SQUAT

The hands can rest on the quadriceps. Rebound and bring the feet back together, then jump the feet back out and raise the hands into the jumping jack. Repeat the "jack, in, squat, in" sequence ten times.

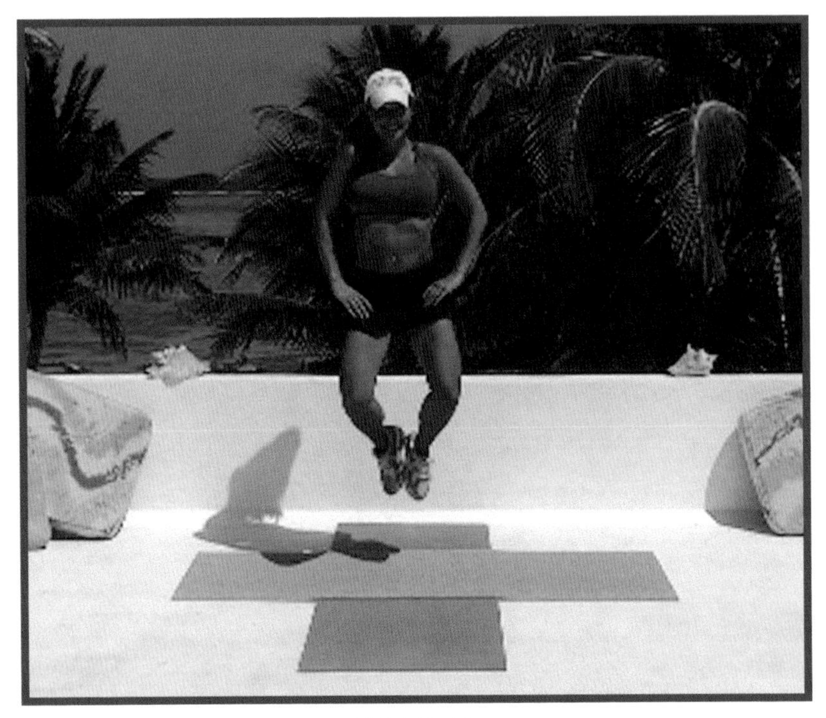

PLIE CLAP

Next, jump your feet into a plie squat again and perform three squats. Just before the fourth squat, you will jump into the air and clap your feet underneath you. The count is one (squat down and up), two (squat down and up), three (squat down and jump into the air and CLAP feet together), four (land and finish, rising up with legs straight). Repeat ten times.

Recover with sunflowers.

Chapter 12

Abs Chiseling

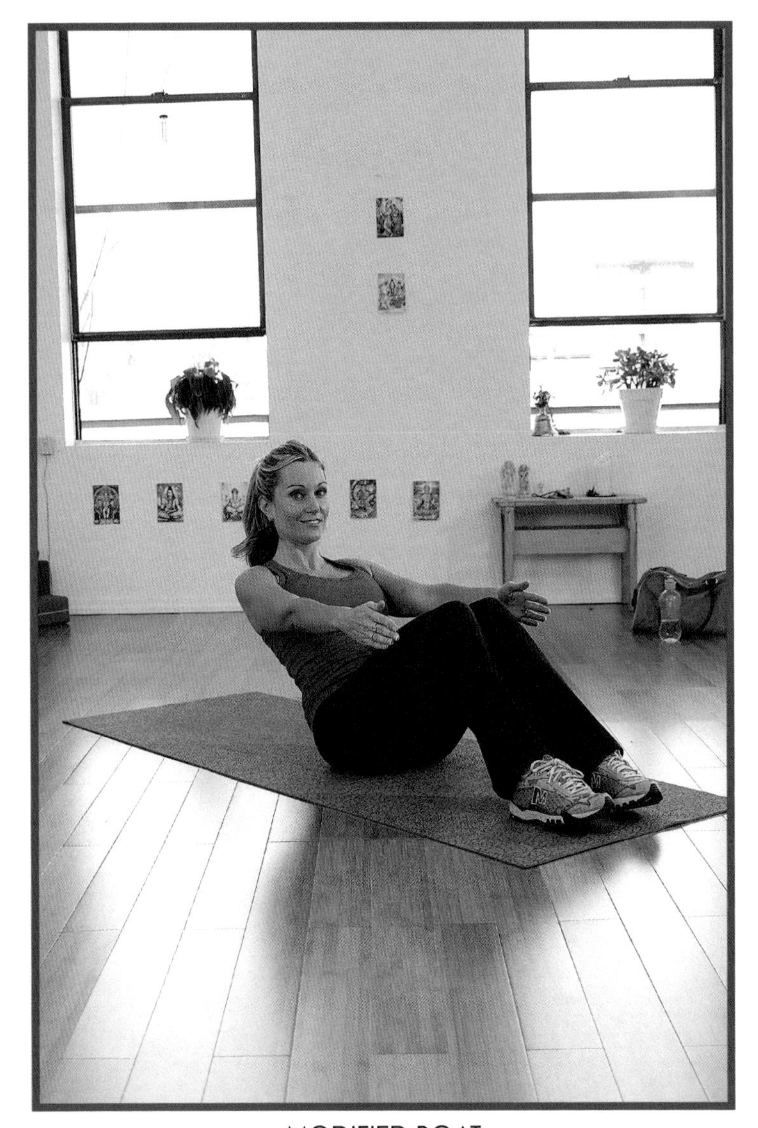

MODIFIED BOAT

Boat and Wide Boat:

Find a seated position and lean back onto your tailbone so that your abs are forced to engage to hold you up. You may keep the feet on the floor with the knees bent at ninety degrees or lift the bent legs off the floor into a tabletop position.

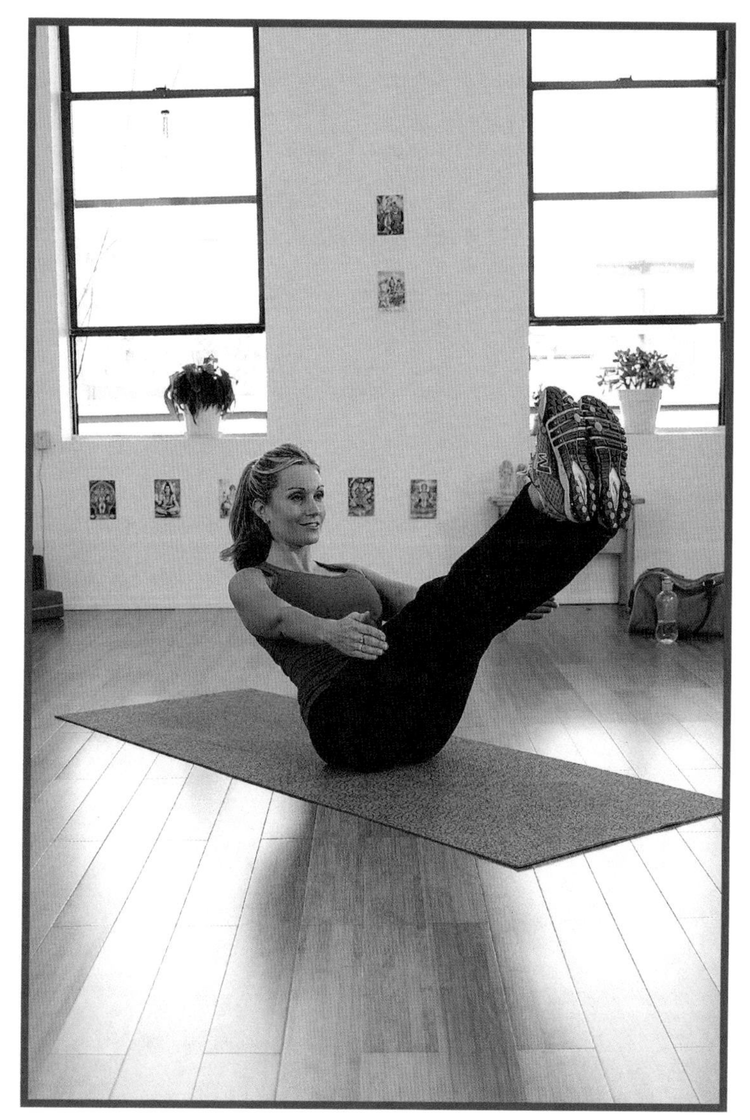

BOAT FULL

The hands may root into the earth, hold behind the knees for support, or extend out in front of you. The heart lifts and collarbone expands as you gaze slightly up and away from the legs. Hold for five breaths and then lower the feet and return to a regular seated position.

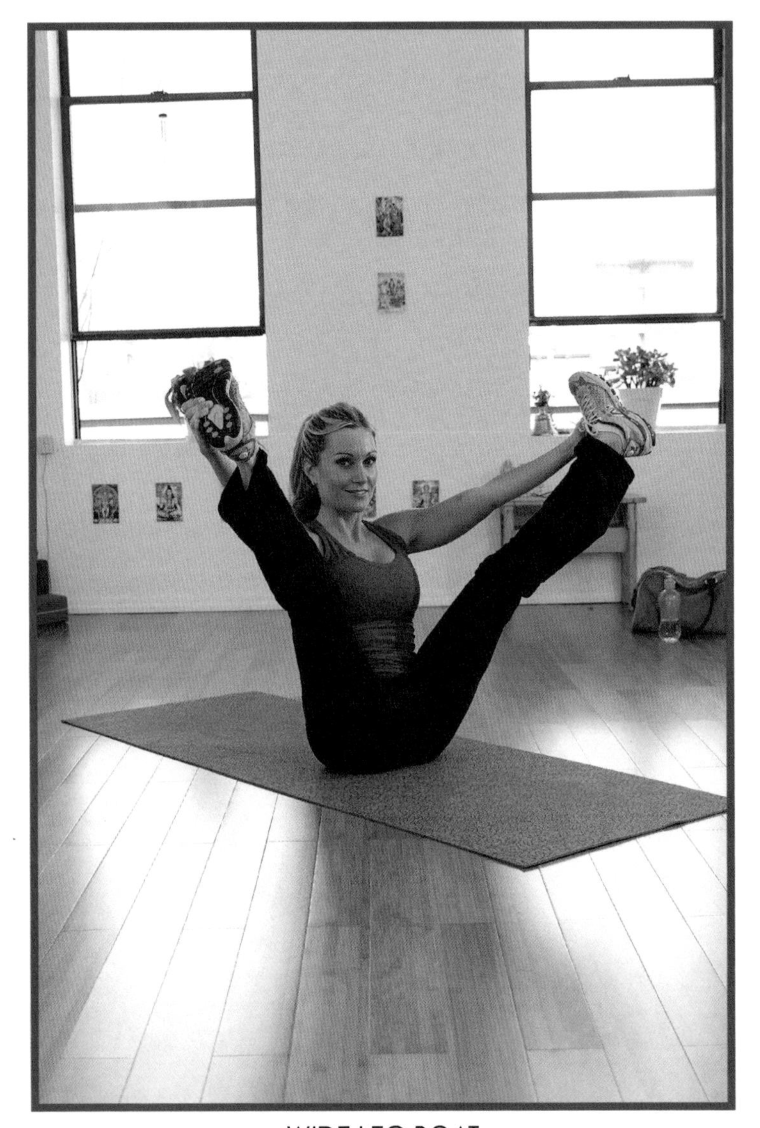

WIDE LEG BOAT

Next, perform another bent leg boat or bend the knees deeper so that you can grab onto the feet with the hands wrapped around the outsides of the sneakers. Lean back on the tailbone again and straighten the legs. Hold for five breaths.

Eight-Angle Pose or Astavakrasana

This is one of my favorite poses to do because it builds core strength, focus, and upper-body strength. There is also a great story behind this pose; it is named after a sage. Check out the book *Myths of the Asanas* for that and more stories behind the poses. This is also a great pose to refer to the video for correct body placement.

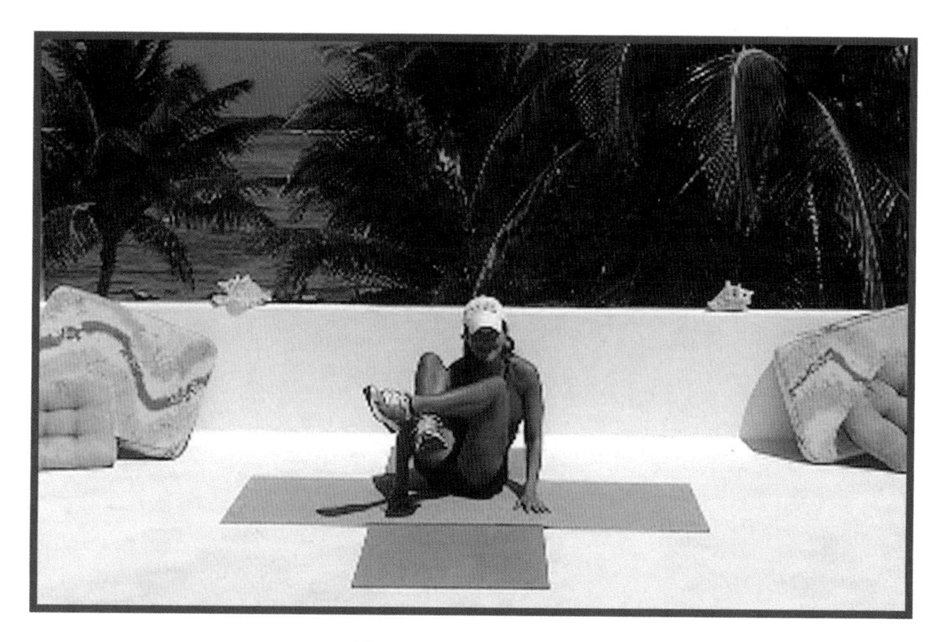

ASTAVAKRASANA PREP

Start in seated position with the left leg extended in front of you on the floor while the right knee is bent. Taking the right ankle in your right hand, place it into the crook of our left elbow and link the hands together. Your foot will be near your left shoulder, and your knee will be near your right. This pose is called "cradle the baby" because it looks as if your shin is a baby in your arms. Sit up tall and hug the leg in to open and stretch the right glute and outer thigh. Hold for three deep breaths.

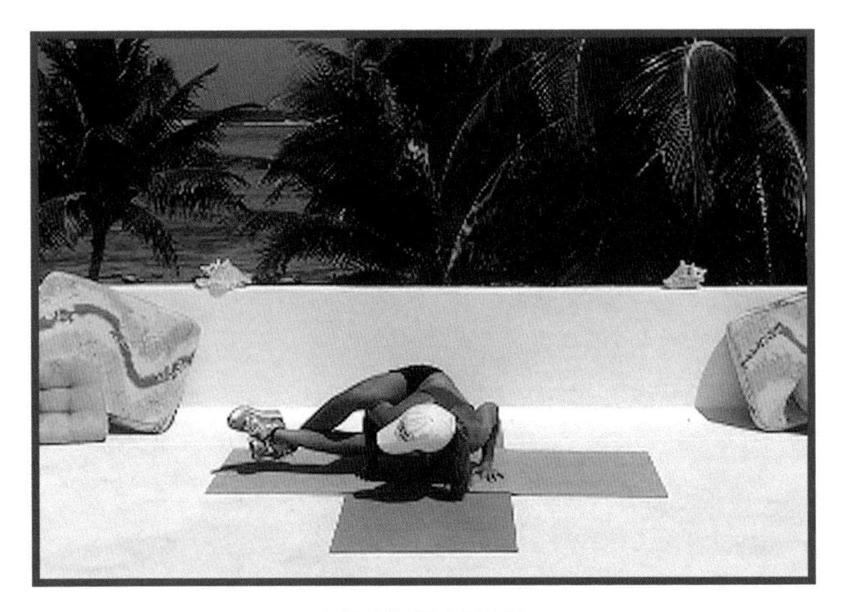

ASTAVAKRASANA

Next, take the right ankle out of the left arm. Lean forward and link the underside of the right knee over your right shoulder. Bend your right elbow and place both hands on the floor. Bend the left leg and link the right ankle underneath the left ankle. If this is comfortable, lean forward as we did during crow pose. Keeping elbows bent and fingers facing forward, shift the weight into your hands, lift your glutes off the floor, and push your legs out to the right, almost straightening them completely. Your right arm will remain between the two legs. Finally, tilt your head and look at your feet, hovering above the earth, feeling strong and capable of anything!

Hold for three breaths. To come out of the pose, simply shift the weight back into the glutes and sit on the floor. Bend the knees and unhook the ankles. You may want to "wring out" your wrists by circling them clockwise and counterclockwise.

Perform cradle the baby and eight-angle pose on the other side.

Cardio Interval—Roll-Up Jump

This next cardio interval starts on the floor so you can begin it directly from where we left off.

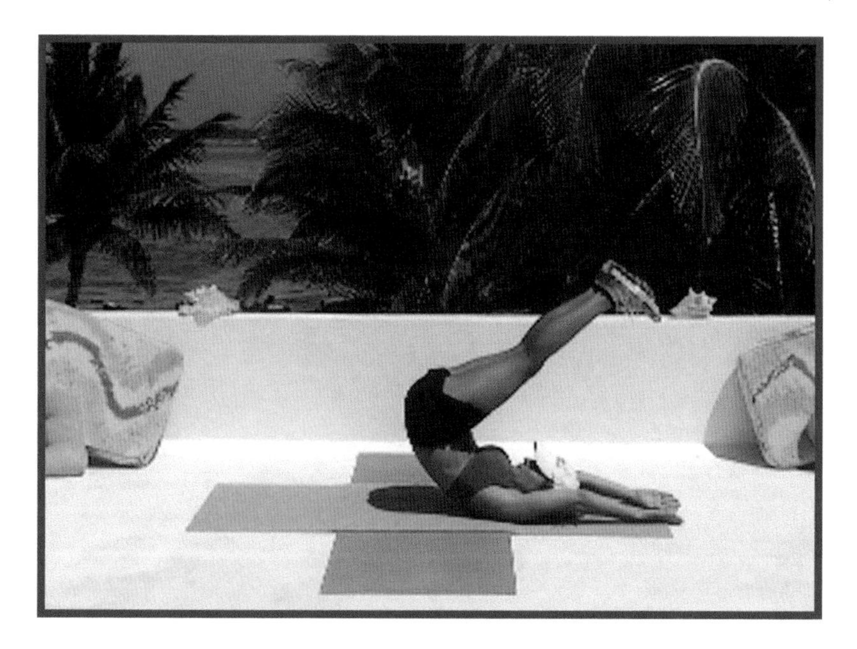

Sit on the floor with legs extended in front of you. Rolling your back into the mat, your feet can lift over your chest and your hands over your head.

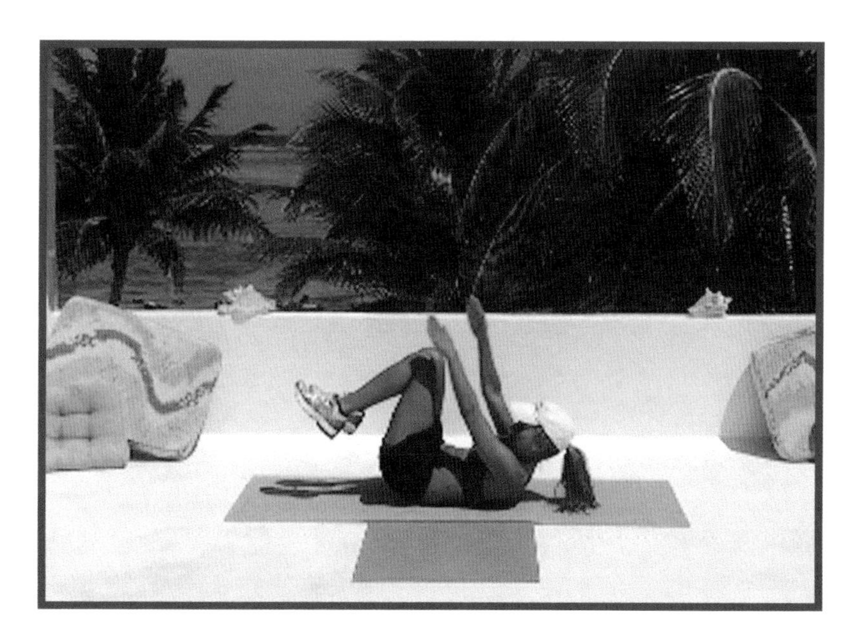

Use momentum to roll quickly back to start but with your knees bent and feet on the floor.

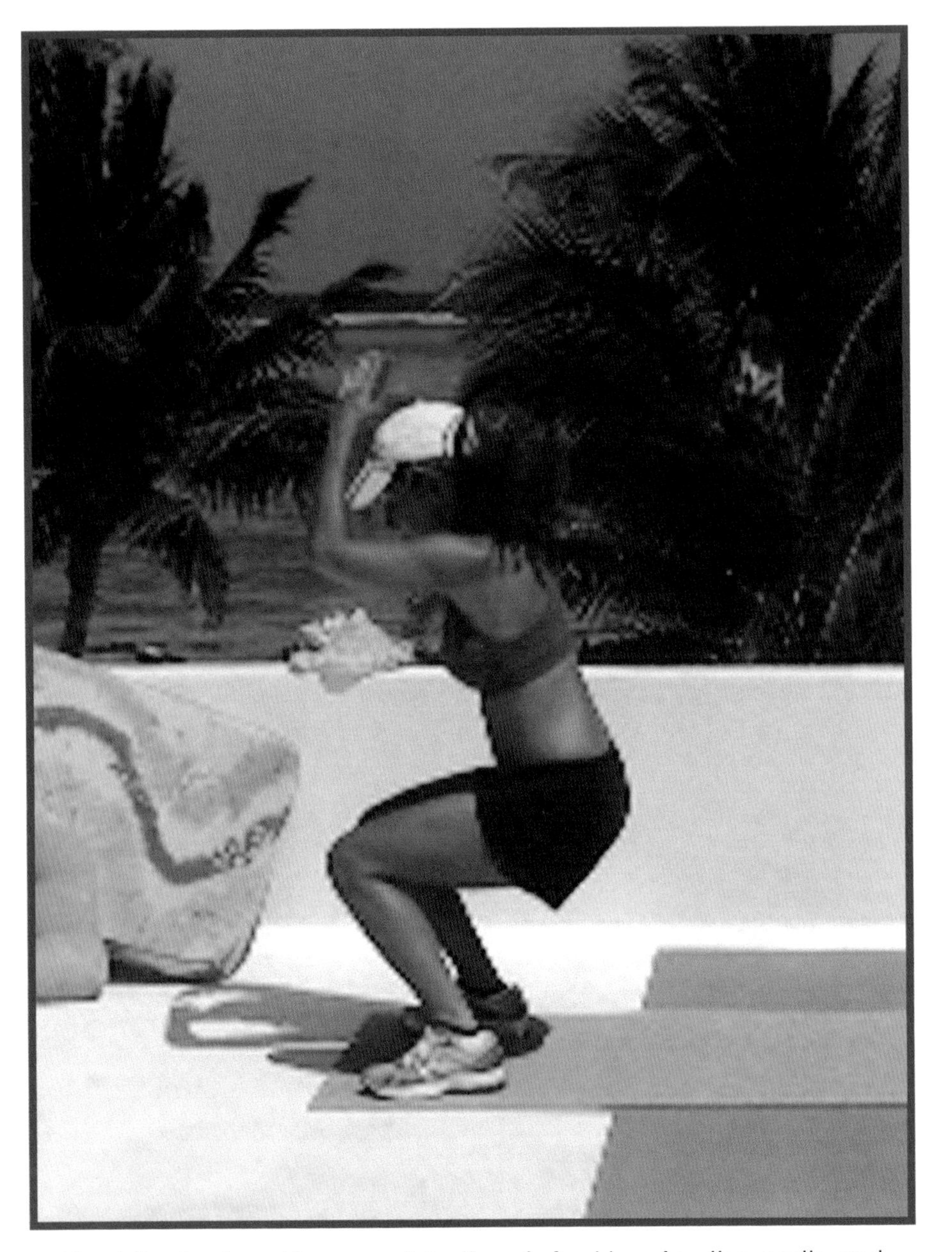

Plant the feet and jump up into the air, feet leaving the earth and reaching the arms for the sky.

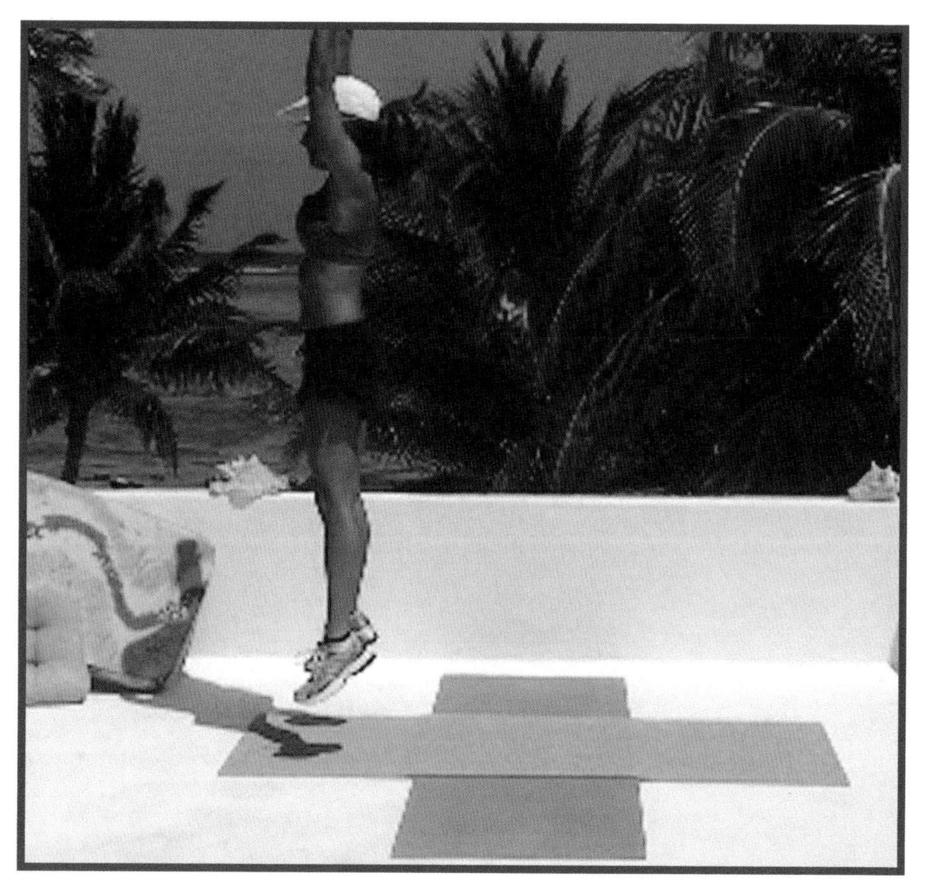

Land softly and bend the knees to lower down to sitting, and use momentum to lightly roll back. Perform ten roll-ups for this interval and recover with sunflowers.

Trainer's Tip: Make it easier by keeping hands by your hips and using them to help push you off the ground.

Chapter 13

Lower Back and Obliques

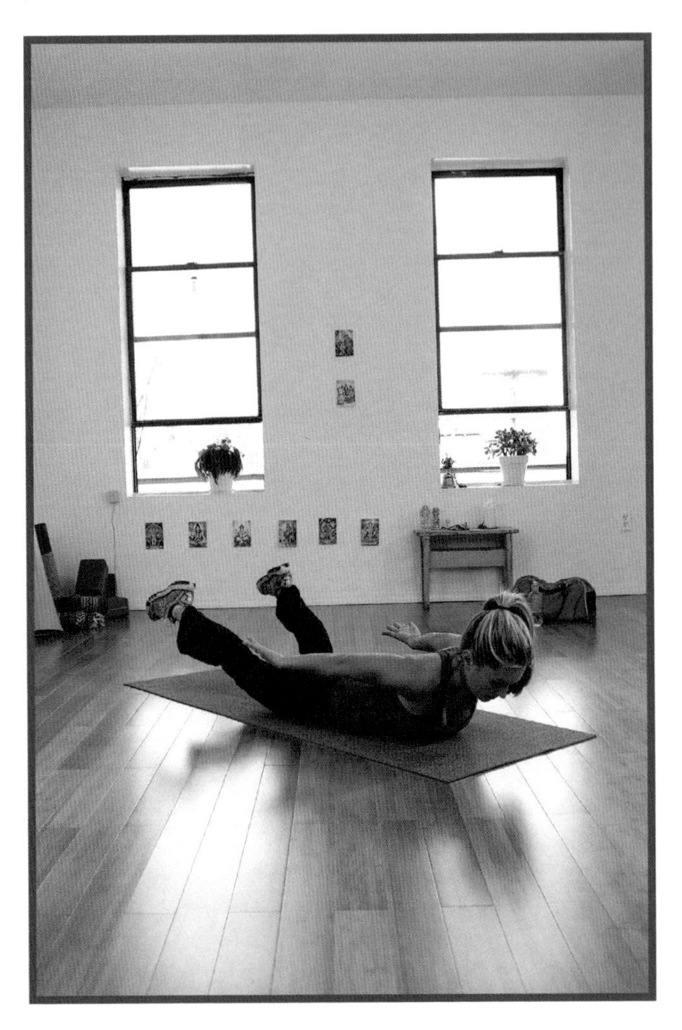

Locust:

Lower onto all fours and then side-saddle the legs to come onto your belly on the mat, lying flat.

Engage the lower back to lift your chest and open the heart as you reach your toes off the floor and hands back towards the toes. The head will follow the arch in the spine and look slightly upwards. Hold for three breaths, then lower the left cheek to the floor or onto the hands folded on top of each other to form a pillow. Relax and breathe for two breaths. Repeat the move and hold for another three breaths before dropping to the other cheek and lowering the feet. Repeat two more times, resting the head on alternating sides. Recover and stretch the back in Child's Pose.

Side Plank Heel Stretch and Thighs

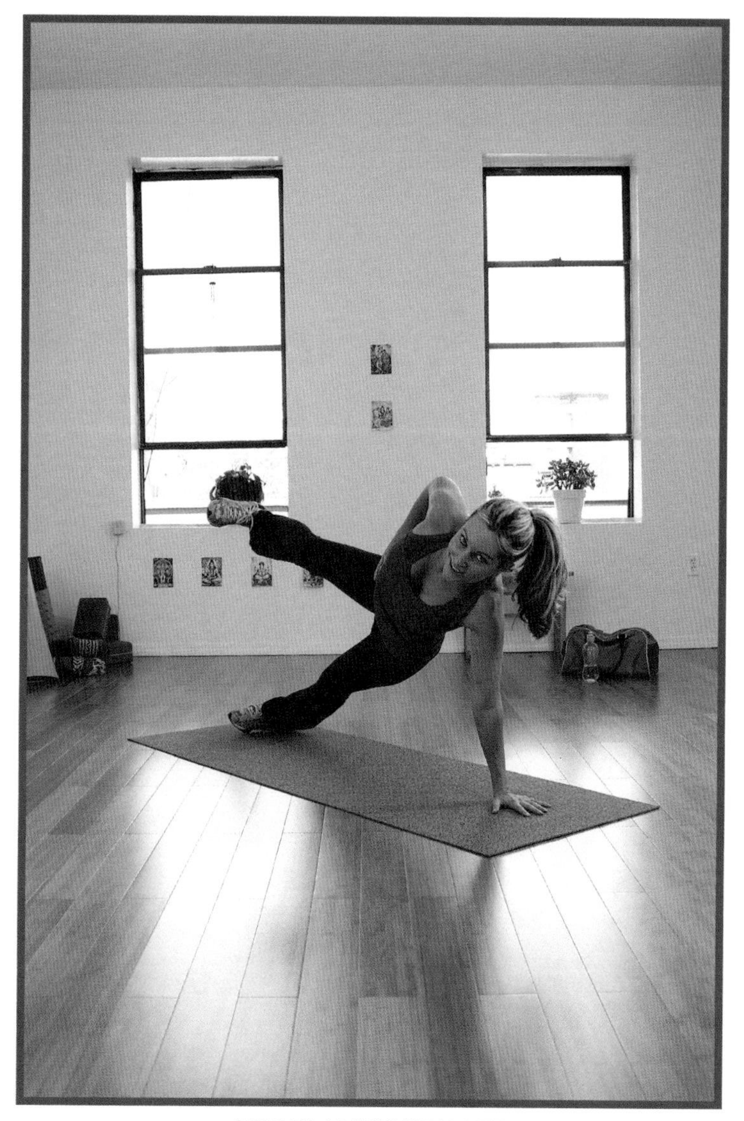

SIDE PLANK THIGH LIFT

Start in a side plank position on your right hand (directly under shoulder) with left foot stacked on right foot. Balance by engaging the arm and core muscles and lift and lower your left leg ten times to burn the outer thigh. Repeat on the other side.

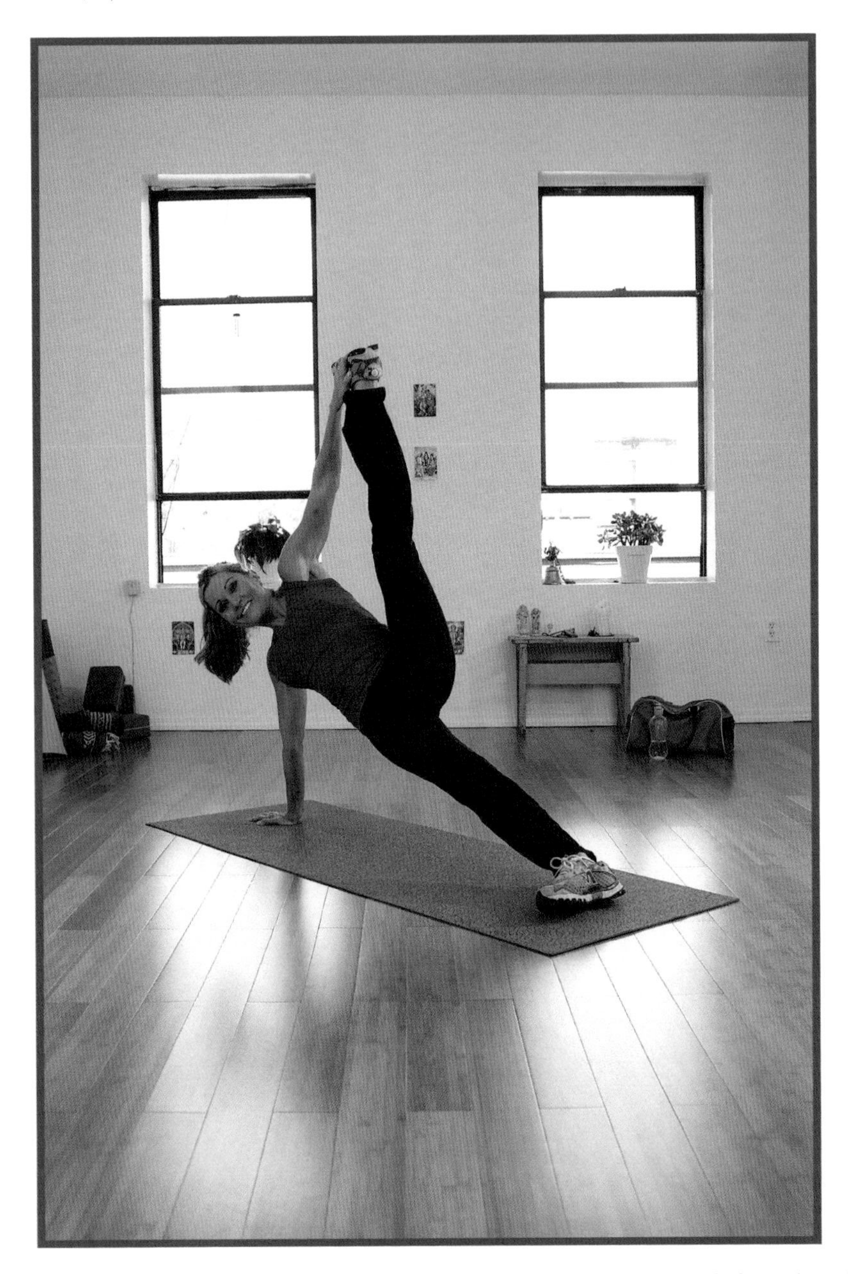

Next get back into the side plank and grab your left foot insole with your left hand. Stretch the hamstrings as you lift the hips and pull the heel to the sky. Hold for 10 to 15 seconds and repeat on the other side.

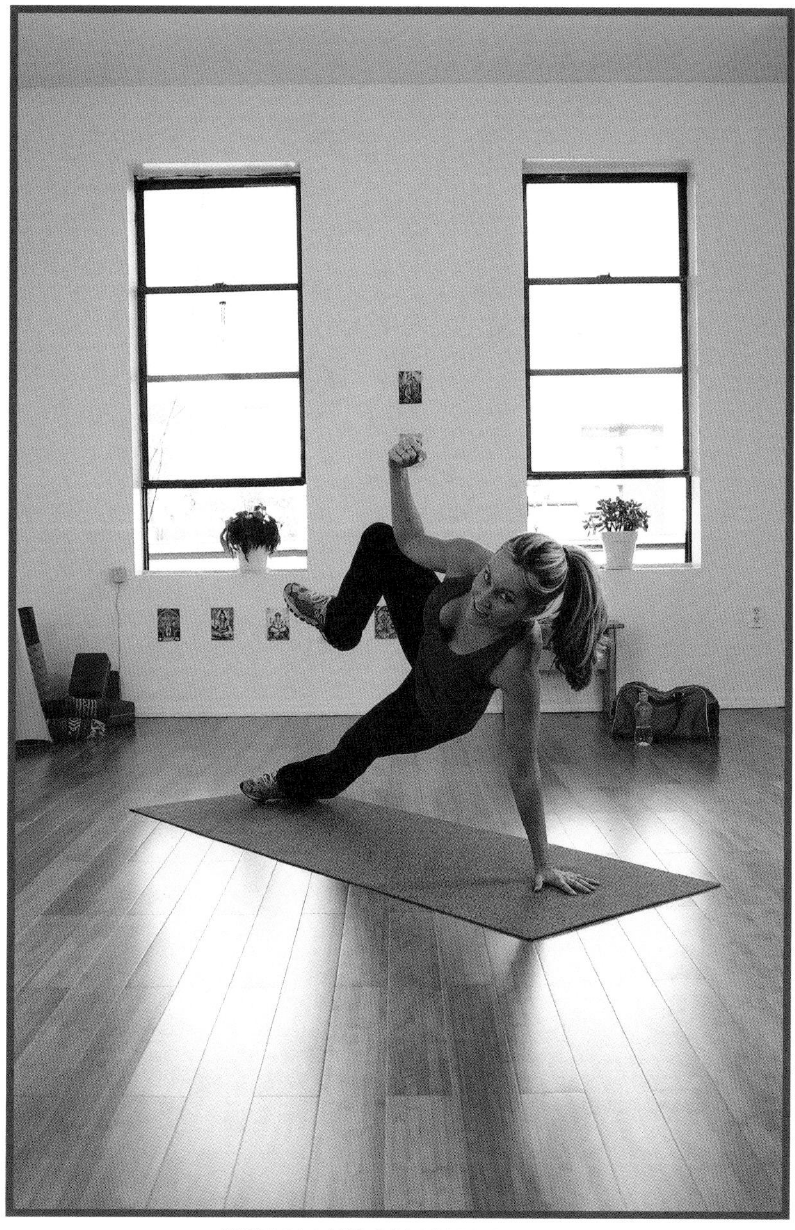

SIDE PLANK OBLIQUE PULL IN

You may also chose to do **a plank oblique crunch** with same side limbs or opposite side limbs as pictured.

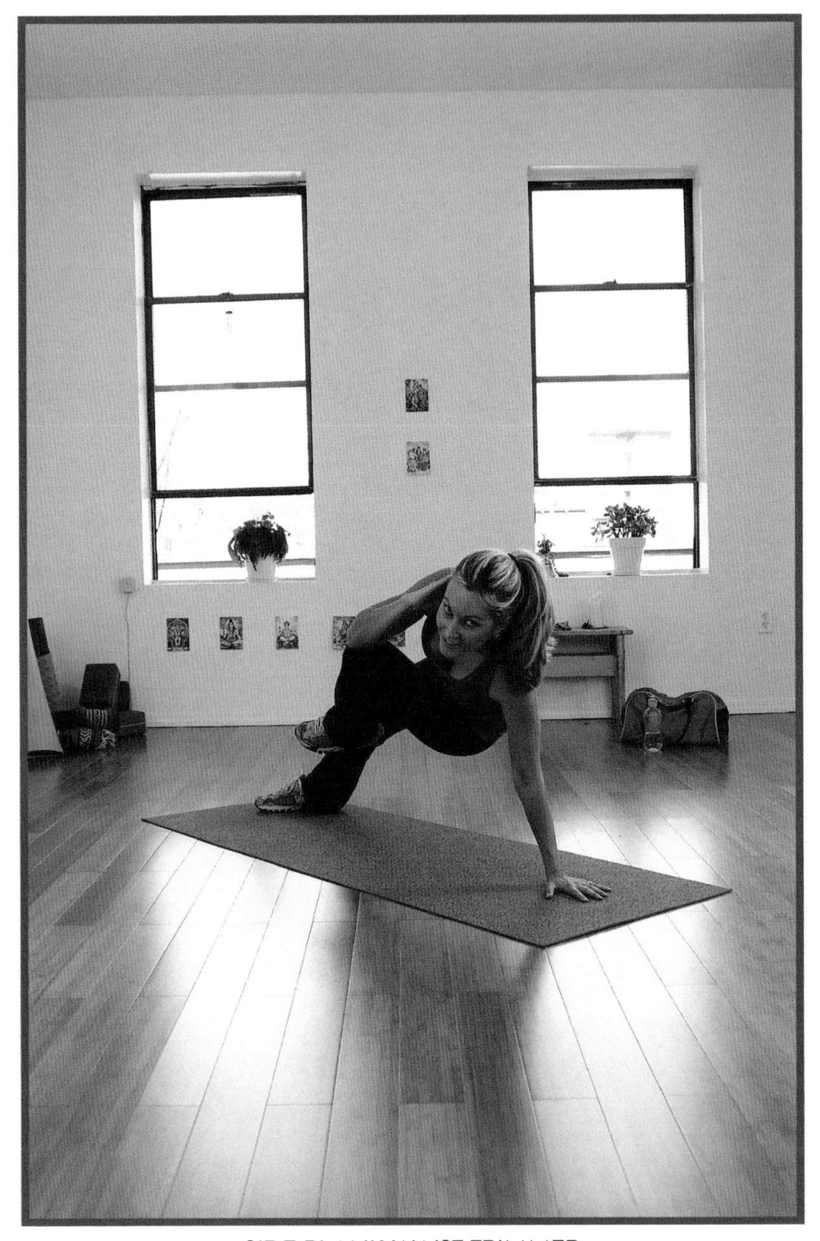

SIDE PLANK WAIST TRIMMER

Cardio Interval—Gymnast Jumps

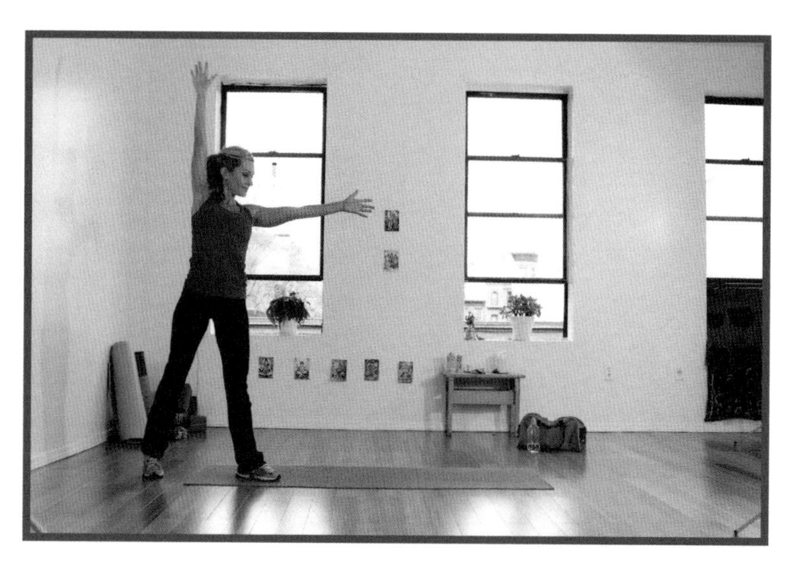

Cartwheel: Start on one side of your mat, standing with the left foot forward and weight on the right foot. Lift the arms overhead with the left arm forward and over the left leg.

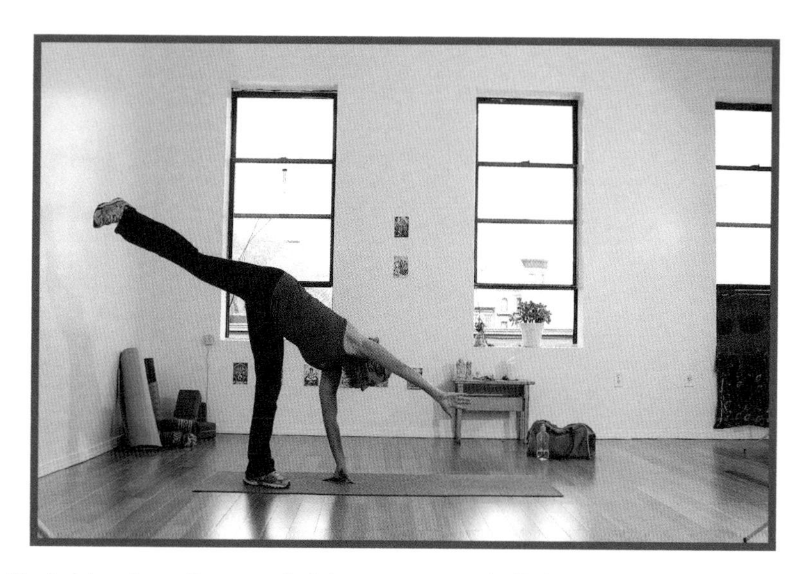

Quickly step the weight over your left leg and lower the left hand to the floor. Kick the legs up in the air and lower the right hand to the floor into a handstand.

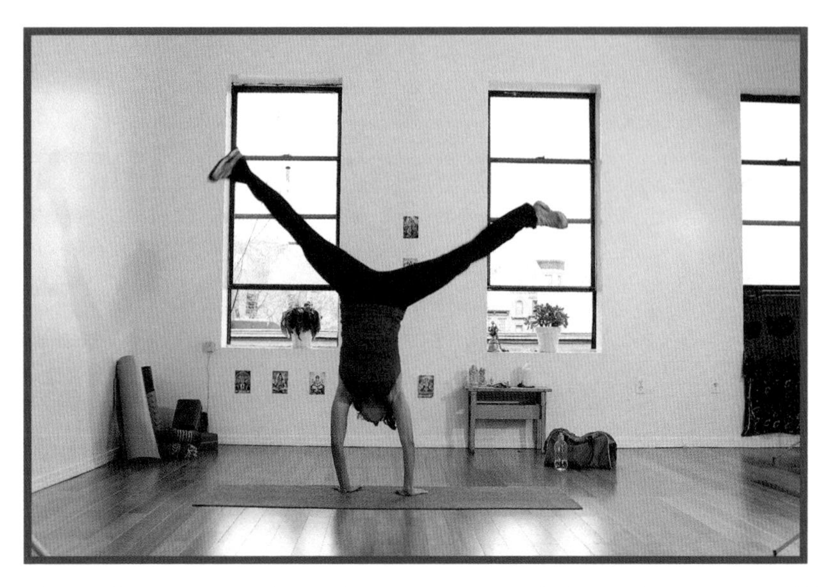

Allow the momentum to move you further forward, shifting the weight into the right hand only.

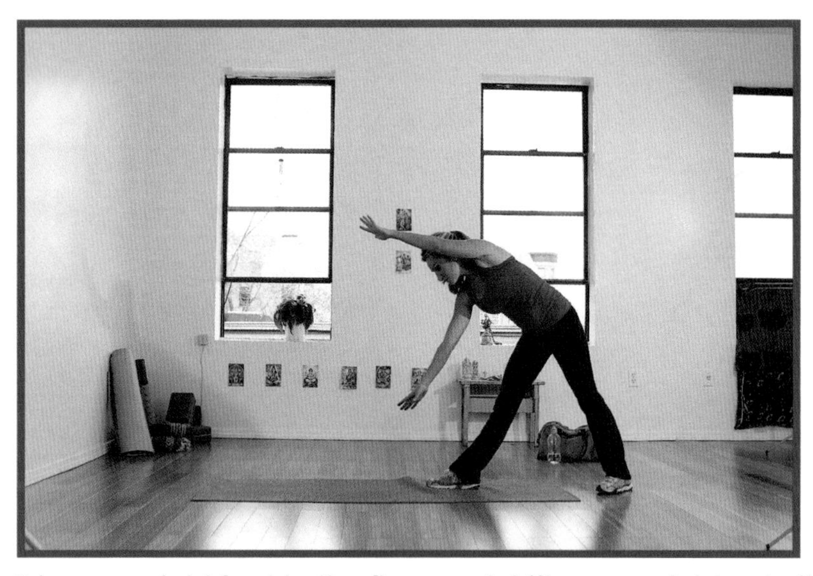

Bring your right foot to the floor and shift your weight onto it as you use the momentum and your core muscles to bring you back to standing, arms up in the air and facing the direction your just came from. Repeat on the other side, doing a total of ten cartwheels. If you have room, you can do several in a row on the left before going back on the right.

Herkie and Horse Jumps: Start standing with your feet shoulder-width apart. Bend your knees and jump while bringing both arms to the sky with your hands in fists. This is what I call the exclamation point or set-up jump.

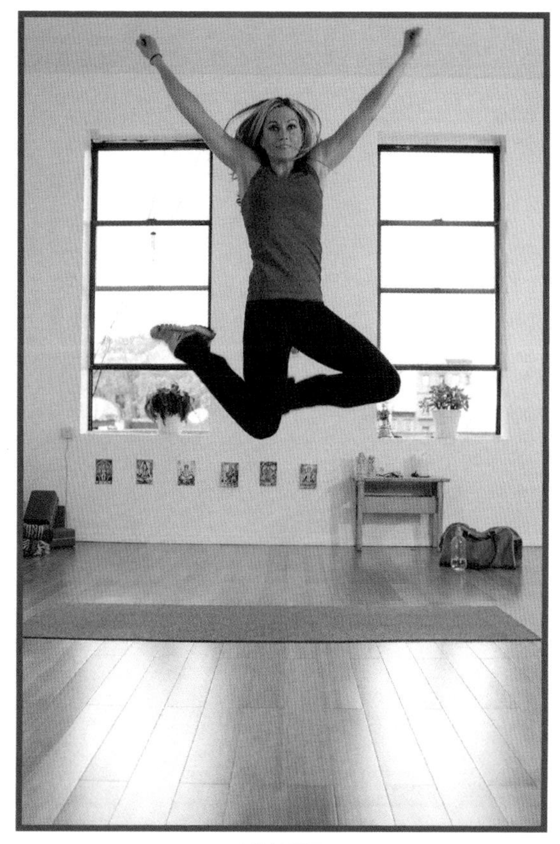

HERKIE

As you come down, or rebound, bring your arms down in front of you towards your bent knees into a quick squat, then sweep the arms out to the sides and up into a V while jumping off the ground and bringing both feet slightly to the right, bending your knees to the left under you and forming a W underneath you. Land and bring arms out to the sides and back to center, lifting them up straight overhead again for the exclamation point. Repeat the rebound and the herkie with the feet going to the left this time and knees going right. Repeat ten times (five on each side). Recover with a few sunflowers.

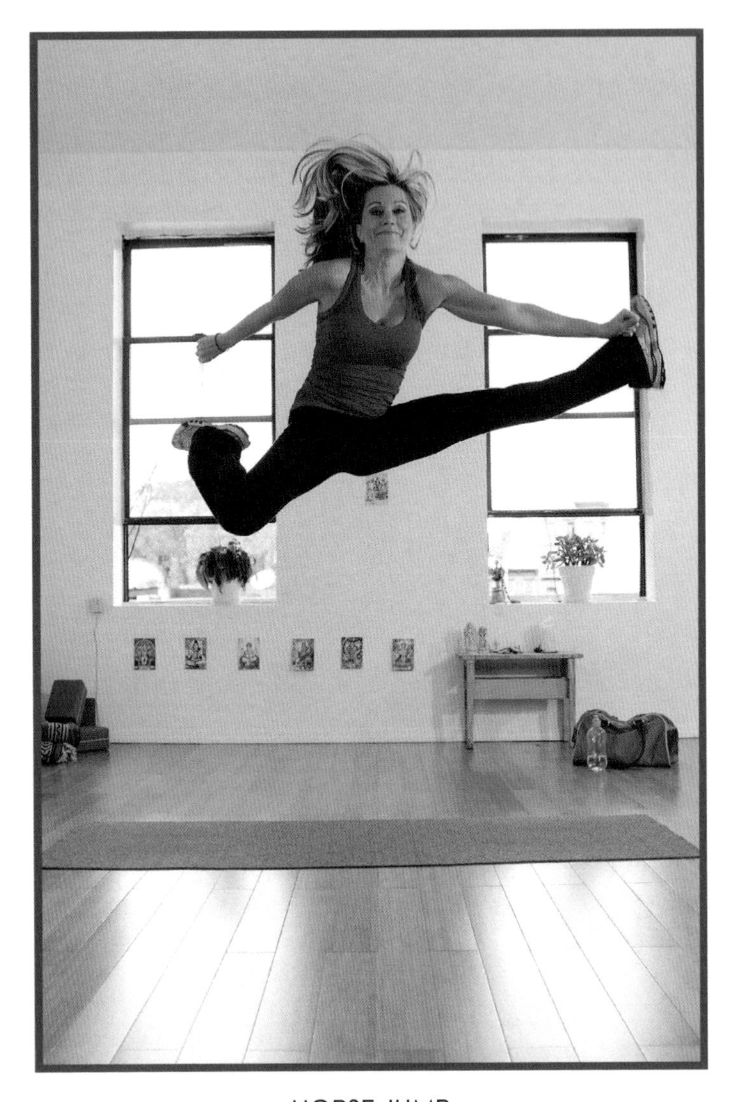

HORSE JUMP

The horse is similar, except after your squat and exclamation point, squat and then jump into the air kicking your left leg long in front of you and off to the side, (like half a split jump) and bending your right leg behind you and to the side (like half a herkie.). Repeat and rebound on the other side, 5 times per side.

Trainer's Tip: You can modify any of the jumps in this workout with a series of quick squats or with spring squats.

Chapter 14

Finishing Touches, Torching Calories with Upper Back and Inversions

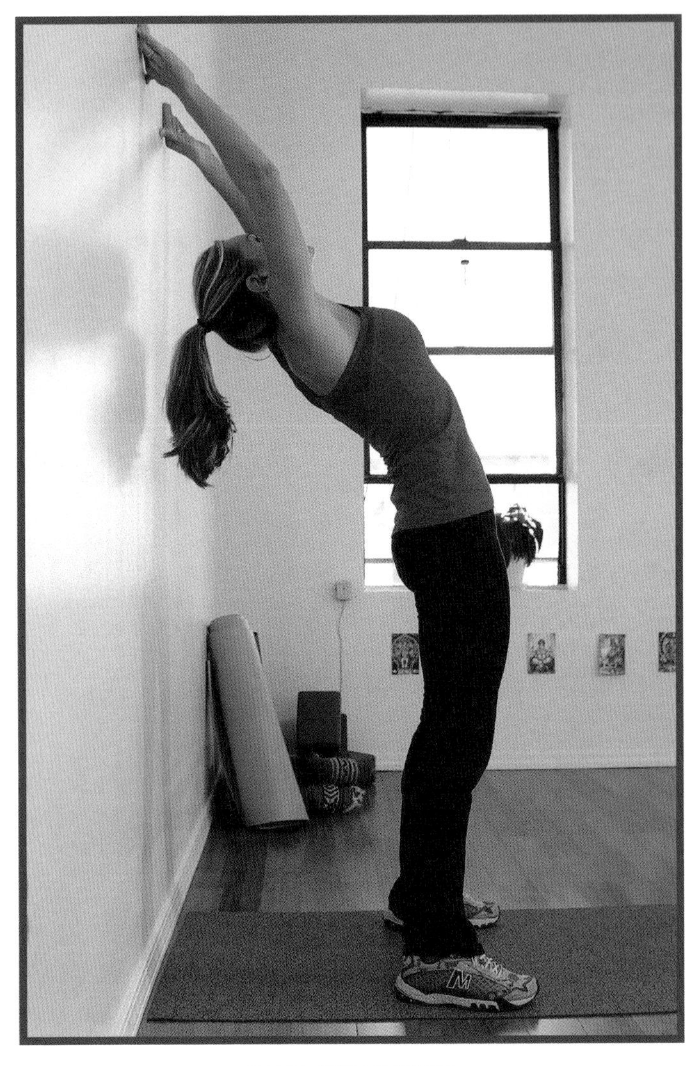

WALL WALK PREP

Wall Walk to Wheel

This is another fun upper-back strengthener, heart-opener, and backbend. Walk up to a wall and step a foot or so away, turning so your back faces the wall.

Slightly bend your back and reach the arms overhead to touch the wall. Return to standing and inch forward a few times until you feel that you could not do another backbend and touch the wall.

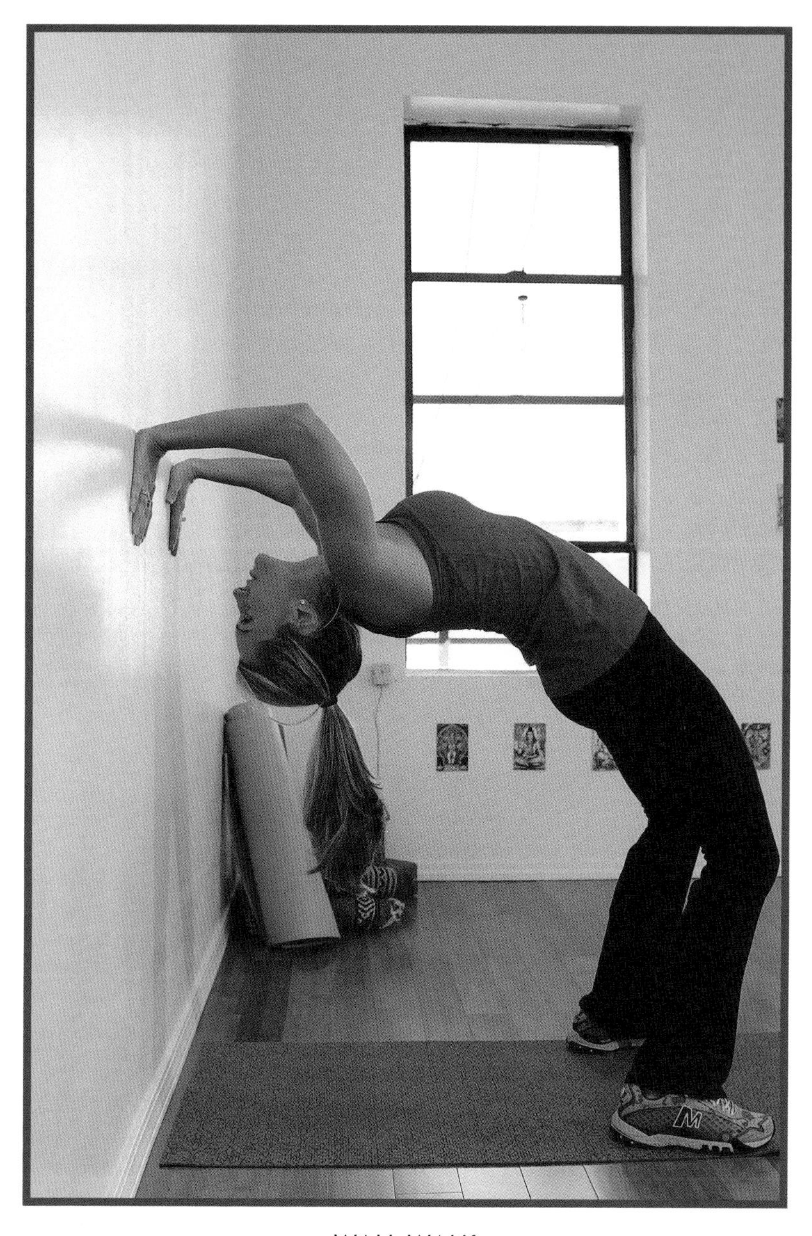

WALL WALK

When you have found your position, bend your back and look overhead, reaching the hands towards the wall and this time pressing your palms into it. Keep the feet hip-width apart with knees slightly bent and core tight.

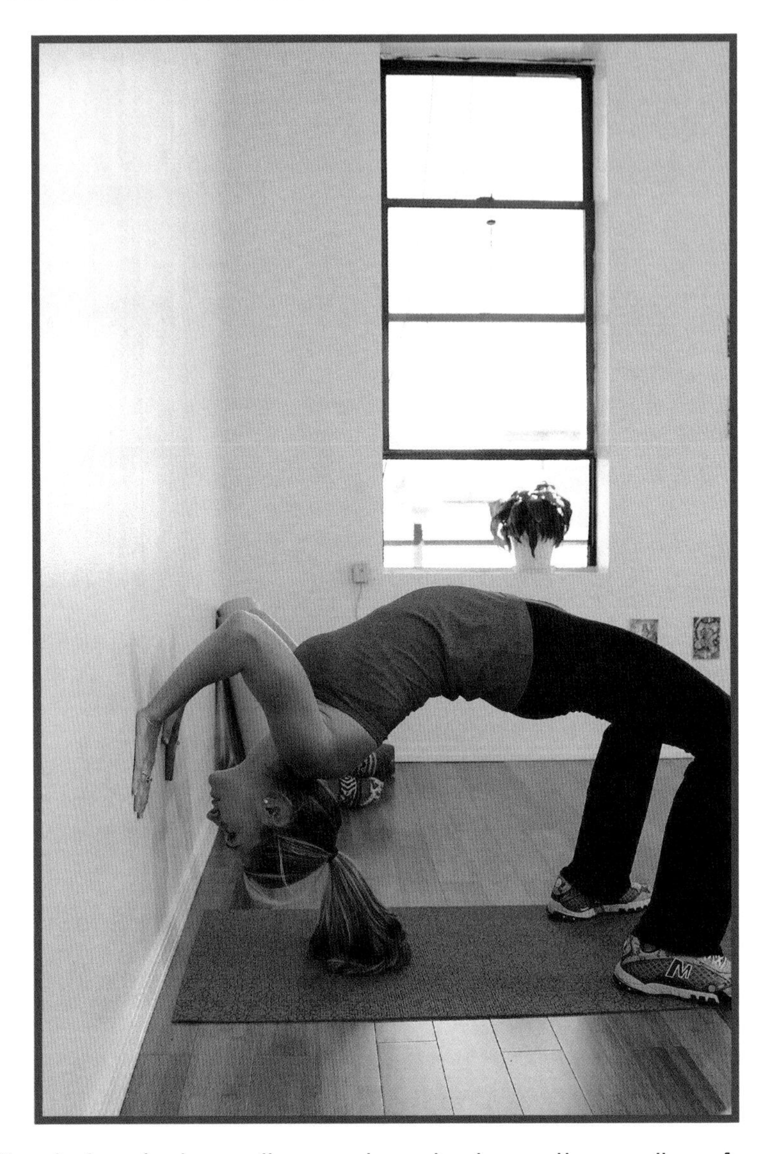

Slowly begin to walk your hands down the wall as far as is comfortable or coming all the way to the floor into wheel pose with your hands on the floor and fingers facing your heels.

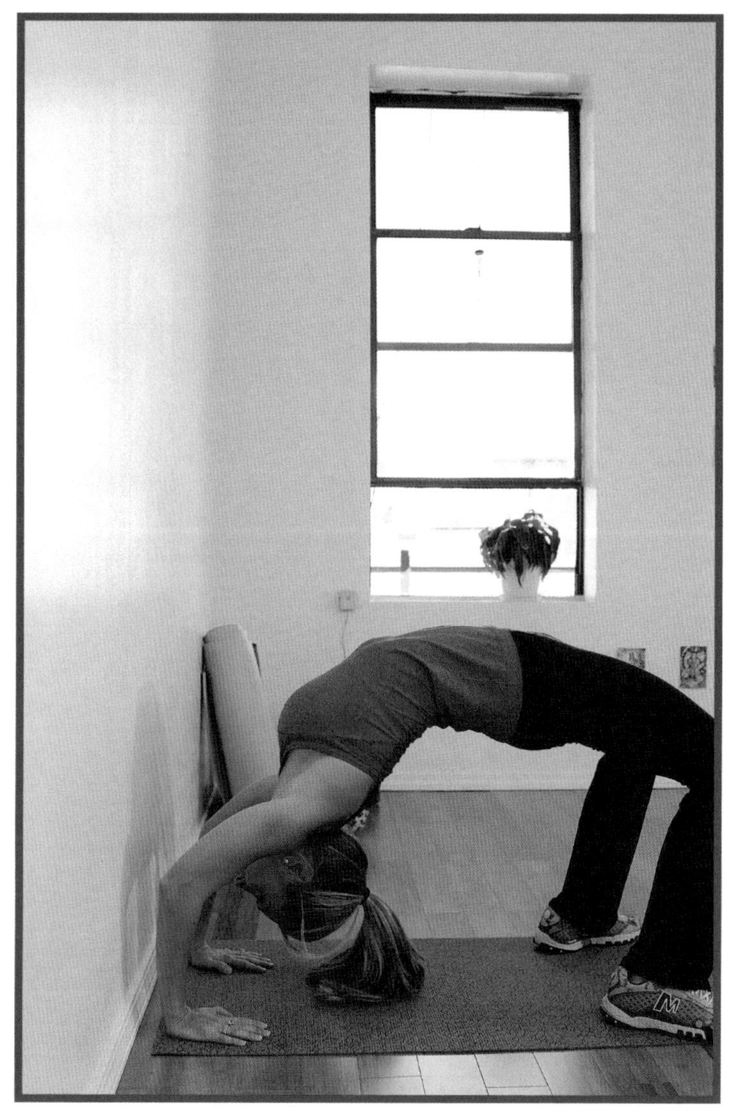

WALL WALK TO WHEEL

Trainer's Tip: Push hard against the wall because gravity will be pulling you down and you need to support yourself until you can reach the floor.

Once in wheel, or as far as you feel comfortable going, press the hands firmly back into the wall and walk yourself back up to standing. As a counter-stretch, take a forward bend and reach towards your shins or the floor. Hold for two long breaths.

Forearm Stand

Another great upper-back strengthener is the forearm stand.

Staying near the wall, turn to face it and get onto your hands and knees. Place your palms on the floor near the wall and line up your elbows on the floor as well, directly behind the hands.

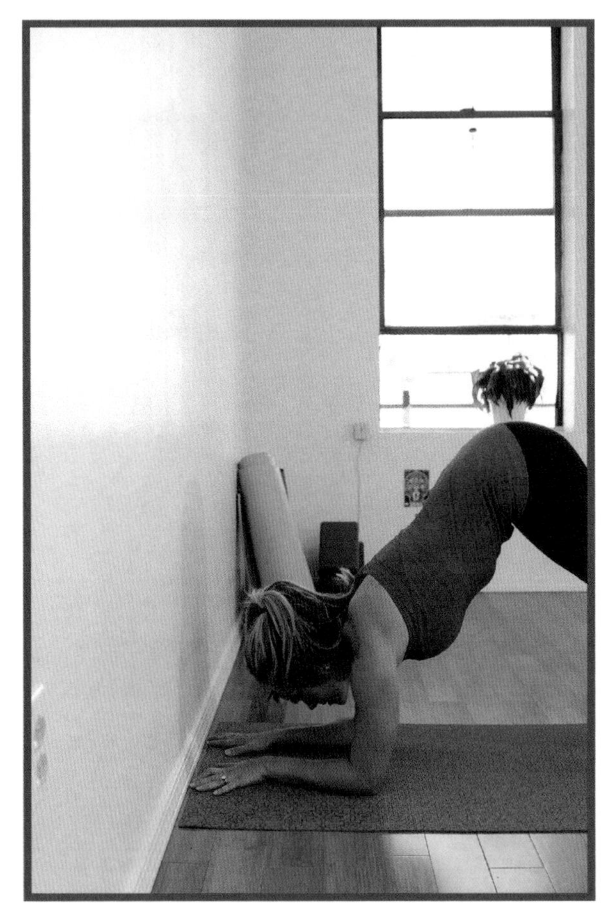

FOREARM STAND PREP

Trainer's Tip: The perfect distance for the hands is shoulder width. You can measure this by keeping your elbows on the floor and wrapping your hands around your triceps. If your fingers cannot curl around your arms, you should bring your elbows and hands in closer until they can.

After measuring, place the palms back on the floor with the fingertips pointing to the wall just a few inches away from the wall. Reaching the hips off the floor, your body can form an upside-down V—similar to down dog and dolphin poses. Walk your feet in as close as you can to your elbows.

It is critical to look at your fingertips, not your knees.

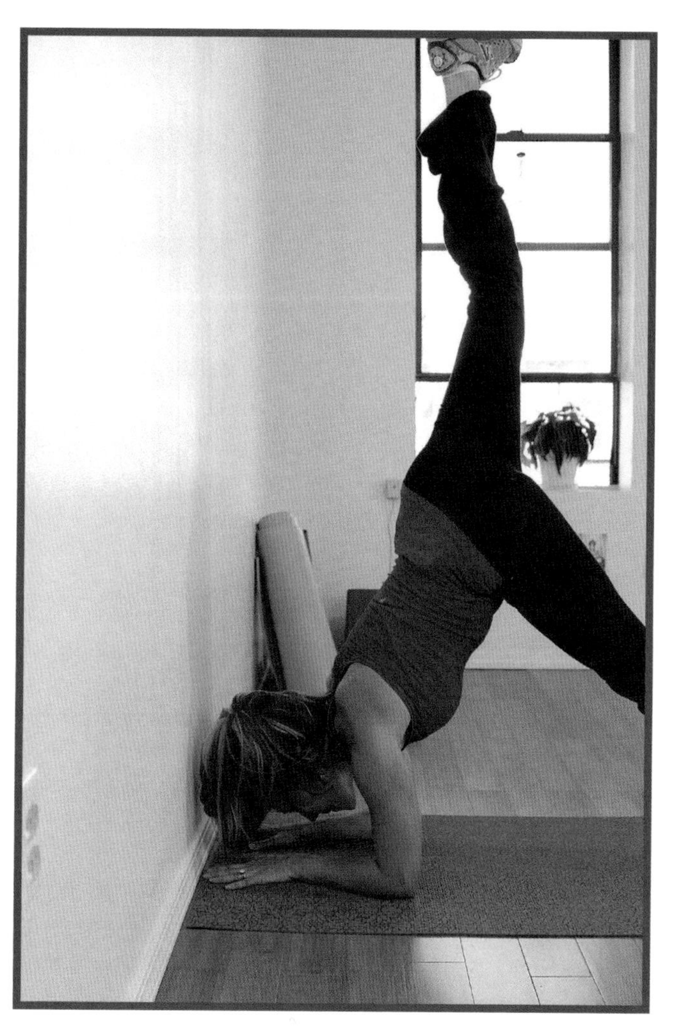

Kick one leg up and then the other in quick succession so they come directly over your elbows or into the wall behind you. Remember to tighten your core and keep looking at your fingertips for alignment and balance.

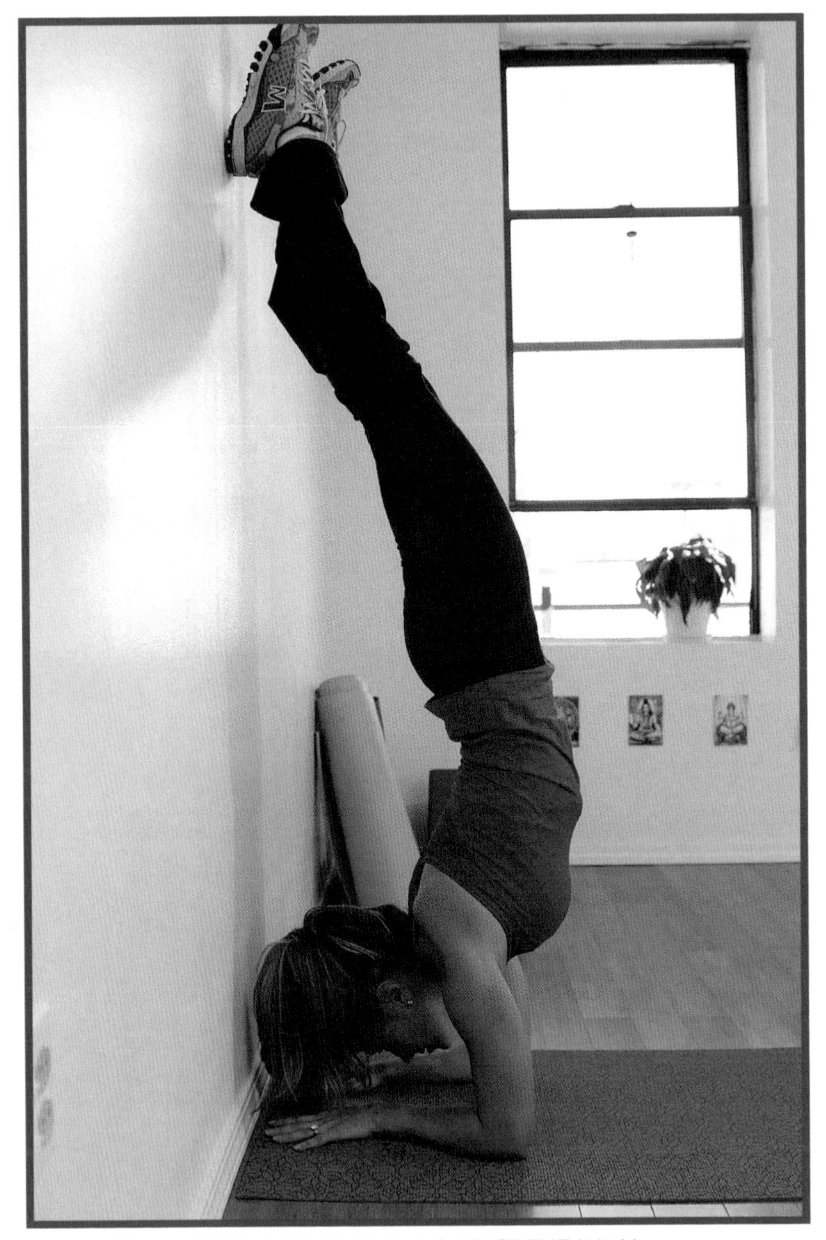

FOREARM STAND AGAINST THE WALL

If your legs are against the wall, slowly bring them away from it and over you, focusing your mind and pushing your forearms and shoulders forcefully into the floor.

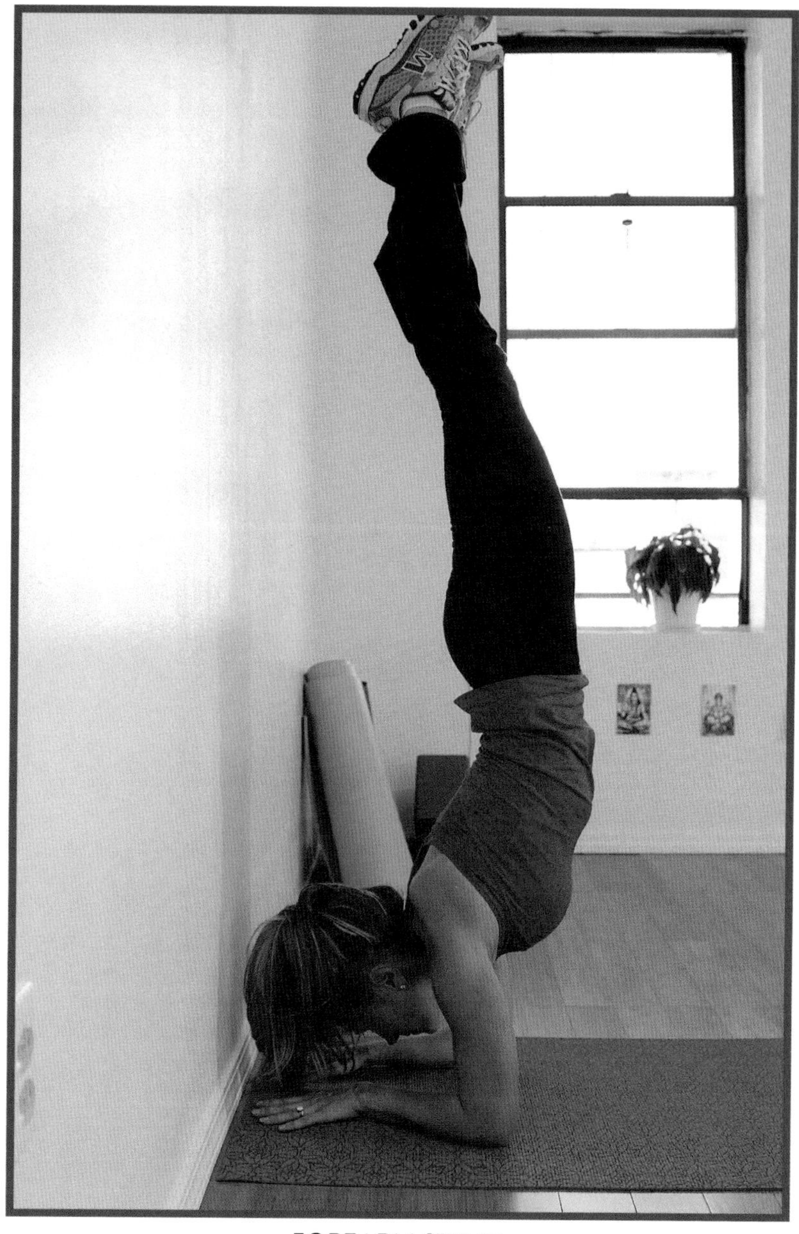

FOREARM STAND

Hover in forearm stand for up to a minute, then lower the legs to your mat and recover in child's pose.

Cardio Interval—Squat Thrust

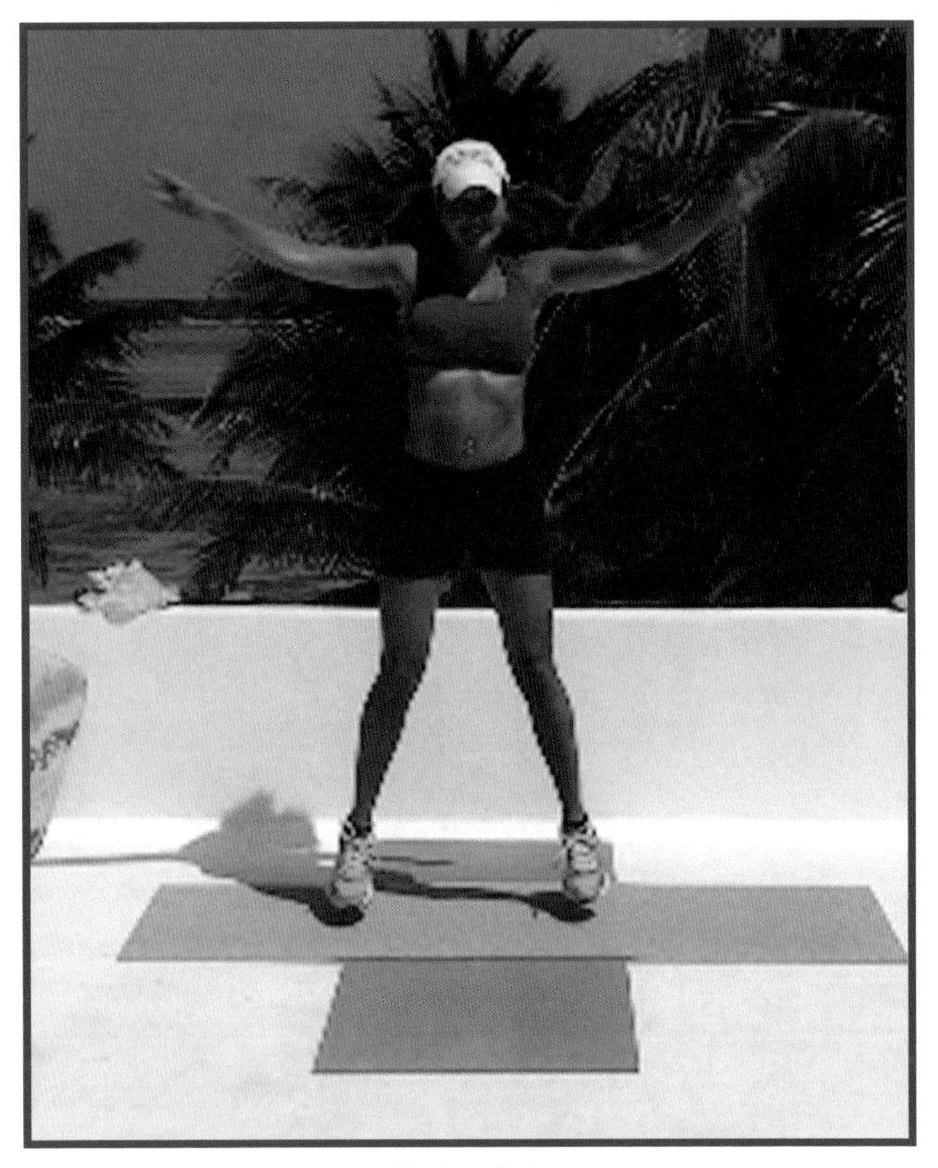

TWO JACKS

This move uses an eight count and is great to do with music. Perform two jumping jacks (counts one, two),

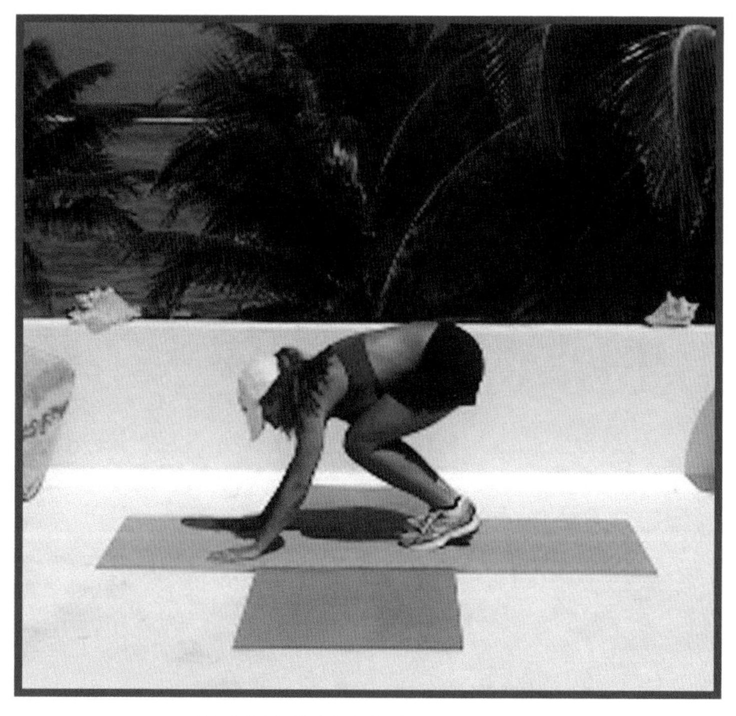

HANDS DOWN, JUMP BACK

then squat toward the floor and place the hands by your feet.

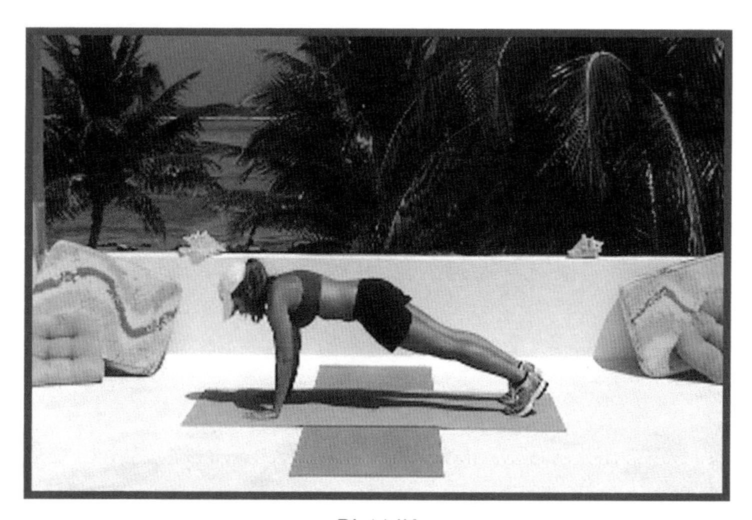

PLANK

Jump the legs back into a plank (counts three, four) do a push-up (counts five, six), then jump the legs back towards the hands and jump or stand up (seven, eight).

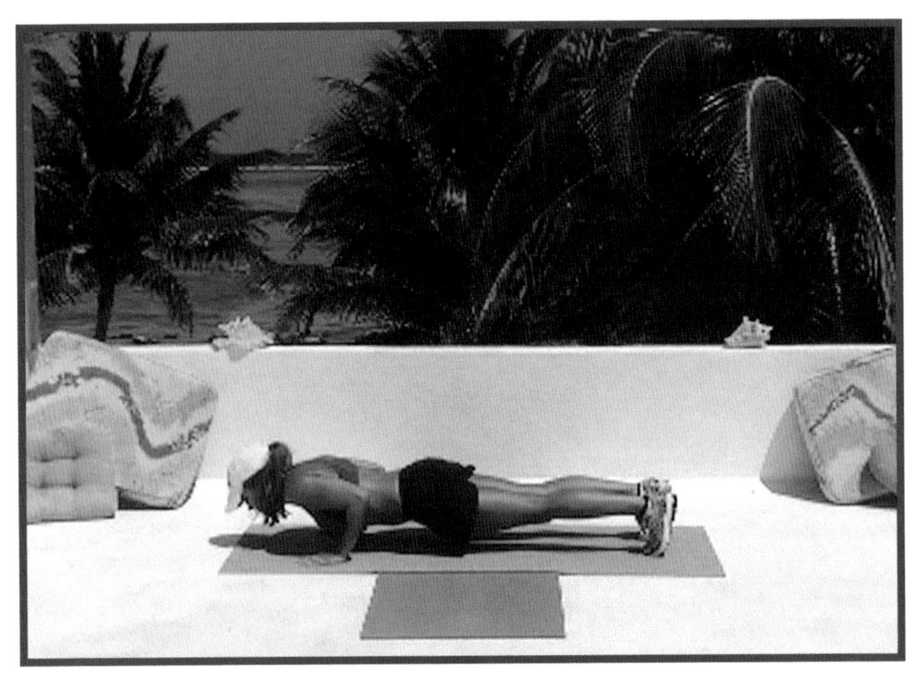

PUSH-UP

Perform ten repetitions: jack, jack, down, plank, push-up, in, jump.

Recover as usual.

Chapter 15

Soothing Stretch (Free Online Video at NikkiFitness.com)

You don't have to be a yoga guru to get your stretch on. Here is a flexibility routine anyone can do after a gym class, bike ride, or strength training routine.

While the jury is still out on stretching before you work out, everyone agrees stretching for about 20 seconds per muscle group after a workout is a must to remain flexible and injury free, to feel less sore and knotted up, and to make your body long and lean.

Some Tips for the Average Joe Not Used to Stretching

Breathe deeply as you stretch, filling up the lungs as much as possible with a full long exhale (think yoga breath). Don't bounce because that's what we trainers call ballistic stretching, and it's a one-way ticket to injury-town. Instead, hold and go deeper into each move as you feel yourself loosening up. Don't strain, but aim for eventually more flexibility.

Seated Hamstring Stretch

Straighten legs out in front of you and fold over them from the hips. Stop when your knees start to bend and lengthen as you inhale then fold a little lower as you exhale and lengthen. Reach toward your feet but try not to curl the back. It is not important to get your head low, but more important to elongate the hamstrings. Hold for 20 to 30 seconds.

Outer Thigh and Seated Glute Stretch With Twist

Keep left leg straight and bend right knee, dropping right foot over and to the outside of your left leg. Sit up straight and hug the knee into the chest. Stay there or add a twist (good for the back and helps digestion and hangovers) by anchoring your left elbow above the bent right knee. Put right hand behind you and twist the torso. Look over your right shoulder. After 20 seconds, repeat on the other side. Stand up. With both feet flat, begin to stand with hands on quads and slowly round the back up, head last.

Calf Stretch with Triceps

Place the left foot behind you, about three feet back into a lunge. Make sure the heel pushes into the floor as you lean on your bent right leg. The right knee should be directly over the right ankle. To multitask this stretch, move the shoulders over your hips. Extend the left arm overhead and then bend the elbow to drop the hand behind your neck, elbow to the sky. Extend right arm overhead and place hand on left elbow. Push the elbow toward the head to increase the stretch. Hold for 20 to 30 seconds and repeat on the right side.

Hip Flexor

Keep the right leg back and wiggle it back even farther, about a foot, so that the heel can no longer touch the floor. Frame your left front foot with both hands on either side. Left knee is directly over the ankle. Think about making the back leg as straight as possible and dropping the hips closer to the floor. You should feel a stretch where your right pants pocket would be. Repeat this crescent lunge on the other side.

Quadriceps and Shoulder

Your left leg is behind from the last stretch. Straighten the torso over the hips again and bring left leg in about a foot, bending the knee underneath the shoulders and hips. To multitask, extend left arm across the body at shoulder level toward the right side of the body. Use your right hand to gently press above or below the elbow joint pushing the left arm into the chest. Repeat on other side.

Inner Thigh Press

Open the legs out to the side in a plie squat, wider than shoulder width. Knees should point out to the sides and be bent close to ninety degrees, directly over the ankles. Tip at the hip and gently press hands into inner thighs, opening up the legs a little wider and increasing the stretch. Slowly roll the back up after holding for at least 20 seconds.

Chest Stretch

Interlace the fingers behind your back and try to press the heels of your hands together, closing the palms into each other. Lift the straight arms up behind you toward the sky and hold.

Upper Back

Basically reverse the last move and interlace the fingers in front of the body. Scoop the belly back and tilt the shoulders and hips forward. Slightly bend the knees and press hands away and in front of you at shoulder level.

Side Abs Stretch

Separate feet again at least as wide as your shoulders. Support yourself on your left elbow into your left hip as you lean to the left. Extend your right arm overhead and to the left. Hold the stretch and tilt your head up to the sky, looking under your arm to the ceiling. Repeat on the other side.

Take a deep breath in and remember how good you feel. Long, lean, toned. Remember that feeling and use it to bring you back to this workout time and time again. Namaste!

Part 3

Chapter 16

Cross-Training Workouts

On days when you don't do the Slimnastics workout, you might want to get some cross training in with other routines. You can check out my other DVDs or the "Shape Up for Slimnastics" chapter in this book for suggestions. On other days, you might prefer running-and-toning routines.

The first time I ran through Central Park, I got lost. I wondered, "How can anyone run in this place without stopping to look at a map every few minutes?" How things change. Now I live near the park, I run there at night, I take personal training clients there for boot camp, and I shot part of my Military Wife Workout fitness DVD here.

But it's starting to feel monotonous because I work out there so often. So I created a revved-up running route using outdoor space as an obstacle course. If your mind and body crave a change of pace, make the park your personal training playground.

Warm up with a brisk walk to the entrance or your neighborhood park or running trail.

Abs: Find a playground. Lie down on the top of the slide, feet below head, holding on the sides with your hands at shoulder level. Keep the legs straight and lift them to the sky to tone the lower abs. To make it interesting, you can even lift your hips off the slide at the top of the move and push your feet into the clouds. Aim for twenty or more.

Legs: Now start with a slow jog on the trail. Run for a good five minutes and then find a bench. It's "time to step up" the effort. Place your right foot onto the bench, and using your leg muscles, lift your body up off the ground. As the right leg straightens, bend the left knee and lift it forward to hip level to engage the abs. Step down with the left foot and then with both feet on the ground to finish one rep. Do at least ten before switching to the left leg. Each week you'll be able to do more.

Biceps and Back: Now pick up the pace and run on the trail again. If there's another playground you can stop along the way for another set of abs, and you can add chin-ups as a bonus. Use a grip where your palms face you.

Chest: Start running again. Find another bench and bust out twenty good push-ups. If you're advanced and don't mind a little dirt, take it to the ground instead. Otherwise, use the seat or the back of the bench, depending on your level of strength.

Legs: Get your jog on again for five minutes then pause for jumping lunges. If you want an intense New York-style move, this is it. Twenty jumping lunges starting with right foot forward, knee over ankle, and feet about a leg's distance apart. As you literally jump to switch legs scissor-style, get some air in the center of the move—what we trainers call plyometrics. You're strengthening your legs and lessening jogging jiggle while boosting the booty with this move.

(If you're doing a loop, turn around now to start back.)

Triceps: Now shake it out, hit a water fountain, and run again. The next time you see a bench, place your hands and knuckles forward at the edge of the seat. Straighten your legs so you balance on your heels and lift your backside off the bench. Lower your hips down toward the ground until your elbows point directly behind you at a ninety-degree bend (pictured). Do twenty to thirty dips.

Trainer's Tip: The slower you go the harder these will be. Also, do extra bicep curls at home or at the gym at some point this week with weights or tubing to work the opposing muscle.

Cardio Interval Intensity: After your triceps dips, find some the stairs. You can do this once or several times depending on how much time and energy you have and what your running route looks like. If you don't find stairs to do sprints, just start regular running intervals, one minute fast and one slow, or sprint during the chorus of the song you are listening to in your headphones.

You're now almost back, so time for the...

Upper Back: If you don't find a place to lie down between here and the end of your route, then save this move for when you get home and skip right to outdoor leg stretching. If you're like me and don't mind lying down in the grass after a sweaty workout, then go chest down and place your arms extended to the sides, forming the letter T. Lift the shoulders, hands, elbows, knees, and feet off the ground, focusing on squeezing the shoulder blades together and strengthening your lower back. You'll also feel your glutes and hamstrings working. Keep looking at the ground to keep the neck in line with the spine. Do twenty of these to work the opposing muscles and even out the push-ups.

Stretch: If you like to stretch outside, do it here. If at home, you can check out the free 4-minute stretch video. When it's over, you not only had a nice long run, but with toning moves along the way, you boosted your fat burn and your metabolism. The whole routine helps me focus on what circuit is next and not on which mile I'm on.

Remember, it's bad to get lost in the park, but good to get lost in your workout.

Treadmill Tricks

Sometimes the weather does not cooperate for an outdoor run, so instead of skipping it, sweat in the comfortable air inside on the treadmill!

Too boring, you say? I have the antidote: action on the machine.

Minutes 1 to 3 (Warm-Up): Walk at 1.5 incline and speed of 3.5.

Minutes 3 to 6 (Steady State): Jog at same incline at speed of 6.

Minutes 5 to 15 (Intervals!): Run one minute at 7.5 fast interval and one minute at 5.5 recovery interval. Repeat several times.

Minutes 15 to 27 (Toning): Walking uphill forward sculpts the glutes and calves; whole backward tones your quads! Set uphill incline at 15 (as high as it goes) and speed at 3. Walk forward for 2 minutes. If you are coordinated and feel strong enough to try this (I take no responsibility for tripping!) LOWER speed to 2 and turn around while steadying yourself on the handles. Walk uphill backwards and pick your feet up high to avoid tripping. It will feel faster than the speed reads, so I encourage starting at a low speed and increasing it only if you want more of a challenge. Do this for 2 minutes (or 100 steps—don't turn your neck around to look at treadmill clock, you could lose your balance).

Turn back around and repeat faster forward uphill walk and slower *backwards uphill* walk several times.

Minutes 27 to 30 (Cool Down): Lower speed to 2.5. Follow with a stretch of your calves, quads, hamstrings, glutes, and hip flexors. (There is a free 5-minute stretch video at www.YouTube.com/NikkiFitness).

Down and Dirty

What if you are traveling? All you need to remember is my **MAGIC ONE-COMBO ROUTINE!**

It's Called "Down and Dirty"

This combo move fits great with any workout song because it is set to four counts of eight…the normal thirty-two beat count that workout songs go by!

- **First eight count:** Start off with two lunges. If you want to make it more challenging do four jumping lunges. (This works the glutes and quads while getting the heart pumping.)
- **Second eight count:** Burpee/Squat Thrust by placing hands down on the floor next to your feet and jumping back into a plank pose. Lower down as if doing a push-up, then lie on the floor and put your arms out at shoulder level reaching away from you. (Works arms, chest, and abs.)
- **Third eight count:** Do two lower back airplane moves by squeezing your shoulder blades together and lifting your hands, elbows, head, shoulders, chest, knees, and feet off the ground (your belly is about all that stays down). Place

hands back under your shoulders and perform a solid push-up off the ground. (Works upper and lower back with chest and arms.)

- **Fourth eight count:** Jump the feet back up towards the hands by engaging your core. Jump up to standing with feet leaving the ground and do two jumping jacks. (Works chest, arms, abs, quads, glutes, calves, and cardio!)

Repeat the combo as many times as you can. Lunge, lunge, down, jump back, lower to the ground, two airplanes, push-up, jump in, and up to two jacks!

Amazing! What else can you do that quickly without any equipment to tone all of your major muscle groups and burn the fat over the muscles with cardio? Ask any trainer, this workout is like magic for the number of muscles you get moving in such a short amount of time.

Chapter 17

Frequently Asked Questions: Food, Trainers, Music, and More!

Grocery Lists: Shop To Drop

Q: I work out hard, but I can't seem to change my body. How important is diet and how should I change from my normal two to three meals a day and dessert habit? What specifically should I be buying at the store?

A: Eat more, smaller portions. The trick is to never be totally full and never be totally hungry. When your "tank" is about a quarter full all the time, you will make healthier food choices because you are not starving and craving.

People say to me often with exasperation, "You eat all the time!" It is true. Before my morning run or while watching the news I have some whole wheat toast and milk, after my shower a hard boiled egg, on the way to a meeting I am pulling an apple out of my bag. Afterwards I am the first to break for lunch to get a large, colorful salad. My afternoon snack includes more milk and some almonds, I have an orange on the way to the gym if teaching after work, and I order sushi when I get home.

I want to share the "health," so here is my grocery list.

Trainer's Tip: Ordering online stops the unplanned, unhealthy purchases. If going to the store yourself, print this list to take with you and eat beforehand.

Produce Aisle: Try to buy organic sweet potatoes, lemons, oranges, apples (the perfect portable snack that hydrates, hits the sweet tooth, ads crunch, and fiber—I almost never go a day without an apple), bananas, blueberries, raspberries, blackberries, strawberries, peaches, plums, pears, red grapes, red and yellow bell pepper, spinach, broccoli, kale, mushrooms, asparagus, tomatoes, edamame, parsley, basil, parsley, carrots, avocado (good fat), oranges (not OJ), leaks, low-sodium vegetable juice.

Bread and Pasta Aisle: Whole grain English muffins, blueberry whole grain waffles, fiber cereal, brown rice, whole wheat pasta, whole wheat bread, whole wheat pitas.

Calcium: Chocolate soy, almond, rice or cow's milk for chocolate cravings, fat free milk, yogurt. If you have to eat cheese, choose skim mozzarella.

Protein: Free-range brown eggs, tofu, salmon, white fish filets, local free-range chicken, lentils and beans, almonds, walnuts, sesame seeds.

Other: Honey, black tea, green tea, balsamic vinegar, ginger, garlic, red wine in moderation, olive oil in moderation, cinnamon, fat free Italian dressing.

You'll notice that these foods also show up in healthy eating articles about fighting diseases like cancer, increasing energy, helping your complexion and hair health, and a number of other benefits. If you have to miss a workout you won't ruin your summer beach body plan because the fiber and real natural foods like fruits and veggies will keep your belly flat. Eat small portions and five to six meals a day. Never skip breakfast but stop eating your last little meal at least two hours before bedtime.

Shop to drop and the pounds will follow.

The Secret Weapon That Keeps Me in Shape: Music

Q: I can't seem to get motivated to work out in the morning because I am tired and just want to hit snooze. At night I am tired from working all day and end up going out for drinks or vegging on the couch. Is there a simple trick that will get me in the mood? When I do work out on the weekends it rocks!

A: Want to know the secret weapon that keeps me in shape when I am not motivated?

A great soundtrack tailored for my mood and workout! Sometimes I put on a up-tempo beat first thing in the morning before going out for a run. At night I listen to fast music on the way home and put it on the stereo as soon as I get back so that I am in the mood for that fitness DVD. Find what genres work for you and mix it up!

Workout motivation is why I don't include standard music on my DVDs and instead have suggested playlists on my site. I think your workout music should be different each day to keep you interested, even if you've jogged that same path, used that same piece of equipment at the gym a hundred times, or done that DVD twice this week. Good music motivates, energizes, and entertains you. Email me at nikki@nikkifitness.com, and I will send some suggested playlists. Maybe some of these songs will energize your workout this week!

Also, let me know what your favorite songs are and I will add them.

Keeping Fit While You're on Vacation

Q: I work hard during the year to look great on my beach vacation each winter, but it seems like by the second day, I am bloated from eating the delicious foods, celebrating with drinks at night, and relaxing all day. How do I stay in shape on vacation without bringing a lot of extra stuff?

A: In the summer you travel to reunions, beaches, and family vacations. Will the burgers and potato salad take the place of your crunches and bicep curls? In the fall during Thanksgiving and the winter holidays, will work trips and family gatherings lead you to airport food and fattening cooking instead of the treadmill and fitness smoothies?

On a recent business trip to Boston, I got up at 6:00 a.m. only to find the hotel gym treadmills full. In Buffalo, NY, during a family holiday trip last winter there was too much snow to run outside and no one wanted to put down the oven mitts long enough to take me to the gym. I had no equipment and no workout videos.

That's why I created my new Fit Travel Workout. Here are some of my Fit Travel Tips to get you through all your vacations with a beach body:

1. Yoga paws. These are small and inexpensive little sticky mat gloves for your hands and feet. I keep them in my carry-on so I can do yoga without packing a big mat.
2. Pack light and organize with packing cubes. They are little cloth and mesh zippered bags to keep you organized.
3. Exercise tubing takes the place of weights without taking up space and adding heft to your suitcase.
4. Wear your sneakers on the plane, train, or bus to save suitcase room.
5. Pack SilverSport antibacterial fitness towels. No washing needed, no odor, and sweat activates the silver ions that keep your workout clean!
6. Double your pajamas as your workout clothes, sleep in, sweat in, then switch. Comfortable shorts, tank tops, and yoga pants work great.
7. Double your sports bras and running underwear as bathing suits. I recommend Patagonia for pretty patterns, thick fabric, and stay-put fit. www.YogaFit.com has the most comfortable fitness clothes I have ever worn.
8. Pack some exercise motivation like fitness magazines, blogs, a travel workout DVD, or e-mail/Twitter fitness updates.
9. Plan to fit a workout in early in the day so you don't mess up anyone's travel/sightseeing schedules or feel it tapping on your shoulder all day.
10. Pick travel and sight-seeing activities that involves a hike, walking tour, or adventure park, such as zip lines, swinging from ropes, rock wall climbing swimming, snorkeling, etc.

And most of all, have a Fit Trip.

Finding a Personal Trainer

Q: I am really serious about getting and staying in shape. I have the book, your DVDs, and some equipment. I really want to cross-train and push myself, so I was thinking about hiring a personal trainer for one to two sessions a week. How do I find one who is worth the money and will bring me results?

A: As a personal trainer, I know that trainers' styles and training regimens vary. And it's crucial to find one who is qualified and meshes with your personality.

Here are some tips to find the perfect personal trainer:

- Ask for proof of certification and how long the trainer has been training clients. Most common certification bodies accepted by gyms are AFAA, ACE, and NASM. The trainer should have a current certification (that requires extra classes, educational training, and credits each year) and a current CPR certification. Also, besides toning and cardio, you may want a trainer who can also do boxing and yoga with you. Not all are qualified to do so.
- Decide if you want to go with a trainer at your gym or if you'll try an independent trainer. Just because a trainer works at a gym doesn't mean he or she is better. Often, the best trainers go outside the gym so they can keep more of the profit and have a bigger following.
- Once you find a qualified candidate, ask for a free trial session. Many gyms and independent trainers offer a free trial session. Independent trainers can charge less if they don't need to pay a gym and can train you at your home or outside. At a gym you need to pay for the membership and the trainer, but research which option is better for you.
- Ask your friends or family members about their personal trainers. Inquire about the trainer's techniques, training regimen, and price.
- Observe the trainers at your gym with their clients. Do they do the types of exercises you'd like to do? For example, do you crave creative moves or need to start with machines? If haven't worked out in years or have any sort of medical issues, you should start with machines that isolate. After a few weeks you can move to free weights to do upper body, then lower, then abs and back, one part at a time. As you get stronger, cardio intervals and multitasking toning moves can be added.
- Talk with the trainer, the personal training manager, or a sales person at the gym about your physical goals, limitations, and current fitness level. Let them suggest the right trainer for your needs and budget or let the trainer refer

you to someone else if he or she is not the perfect fit for your fitness or price range.

- Emotionally, do you need a quiet supporter, a cheerleader, or a drill sergeant to motivate you? Which one will you need to get you looking forward to sessions and push you the hardest and keep you from wanting to give up?
- Has your trainer ever been interviewed in a fitness magazine? Written his/her own fitness-related articles? Does he or she have a blog where you can learn about his or her philosophy and style? Google the trainers or check Yelp reviews to see if their clients are happy with them.
- Ask for referral phone numbers and e-mail addresses so you can talk to some of their other clients, especially for independent trainers.
- Know their cancellation policies. For example, do you pay up front, for how many sessions in advance, and will you lose your session if you have to cancel within twenty-four hours? Many times that is the policy so that they don't save a slot for you and show up, only to lose the money when they could have been training another client or stayed in bed.

Hopefully this list will help you to interview trainers.

If all else fails, or you can't afford a trainer, I will be your trainer through the year through my DVDs and weekly motivational newsletters—all for a quarter of the price of one session. Check out Booty Camp and Hard Core Abs DVDs when and if you need some cross-training along with your Slimnastics.

New Moms and Pregnancy Workouts

Q: I had a hard time getting back into shape after my first baby even though I was super-fit before. Now I am pregnant again. How do I stay in shape during pregnancy and lose weight/tone up after the baby?

A: Where do I begin? I had a C-section and complications afterwards. But I got in good enough shape to shoot a Baby Booty Camp fitness DVD with my baby boy when he was just four months old. You can too if you follow these directions.

1. Keep working out while pregnant. Check witı and once you get the okay, you should be aı percent of what you did before.
2. Breastfeed. Not only do studies show that it is hı you and the baby, but you burn so many calories ı will be waking up famished even if the baby is not waking you. I weighed less after six months of nursing than before I got pregnant.
3. Get into Baby Bootie Camp! I can walk you though moves like "rocking" outer thighs, baby triceps dips and baby biceps curls, toddler tosses, and patty-cake crunches.
4. Work out on the playground when the baby gets bigger—you'll be spending plenty of time there, so don't waste it. My playground routine includes moves like slide-abs and triceps dips, wing plank pikes, ladder lunges, monkey bar pull-ups, and more.

Email me for a Bootie Camp or playground workout demo at nikki@nikkifitness.com.

Show It Off—You Are the Celebrity Posing Tips

Q: I work out and look great in real life, but when it comes to pictures, I still look ten pounds heavier. What gives? I have a big event coming up and I want to look as good as I feel.

A: Now that you have your Slimnastics body, you feel like a celebrity! You might as well look like one in your photos, too. I created a free how-to video that you can find at www.redcarpetrunway.com. Learn how to choose the right dress, jewelry, how to minimize the size of your arms in your photos, how to stand in 3-D for a longer, leaner look, ways to minimize your waist, and, of course, how to find and create your own personalized red carpet runway!

Chapter 18

Exercise Your Soul!

The reason I love yoga class is that it improves your body as well as your mind and soul. You leave wanting to be more calm, treat people better, and be a nicer person...almost like church! Part of this comes from something called *Patanjali's Eight Limbs of Yoga*.

The American Fitness Association of America, or AFAA (www.affa.com), certifies personal trainers and provides continuing education about many areas of fitness, including yoga. AFFA teaches that Patanjali wrote the *Yoga Sutras*, and he became one of the best known yogis while popularizing these guideline for yoga practices.

I would like to share with you the first one, so you can start exercising your soul along with your body!

LIMB ONE: THE YAMAS (Things to Restrict)

The following five restrictions are meant to clear away negative thoughts and actions to make way for pure and clean living.

Ahimsa: Do no harm. This yama means non-violence or non-injury to oneself and others. This idea is central to yoga, as the focus of yoga is non-competitive. The idea of no pain, no gain, which is sometimes part of the practice of conventional Western fitness modalities, does not belong in yoga. Ahimsa also means using non-violent words, thinking non-violent thoughts, and avoiding negative self-talk, such as I'm stupid or I'm fat. Negative self-talk is essentially doing harm to oneself. Ahimsa is the embodiment of honoring oneself and others.

Satya: Do not lie. This yama also relates to self and to interaction with others and reminds yogis to act in complete truth at all times. According to ancient yogic scriptures, the truth cannot bring harm. Being truthful in all parts of one's life creates higher standards and builds loftier character.

Asteya: Do not steal. This yama reminds yogis not to take something that does not belong to them. Aside from tangible items, it is possible to steal intangible things as well, such as another person's confidence, pride, or attention.

Brahmacharya: Do not ignore virtue or abstinence. This yama is believed by some to be more about virtue than abstinence. It reminds yogis to think of others with love and respect rather than with selfishness and lust. This yama does not demand that every yogi should live a life without a spouse or children and be celibate. This yama, like the others, simply encourages purity of thought and action, in this case, in relation to love and sexual behaviors.

Aparigraha: Do not be greedy. This yama is a reminder not to accumulate unnecessary things. Excessive possessions add clutter to life and bring clutter to the mind and spirit as well. This yama encourages simplification and letting go of materialistic desires and envy. Again, purity of thought and action are emphasized. Less is more.

Fitness—fit it in…inside and out!

Nikki

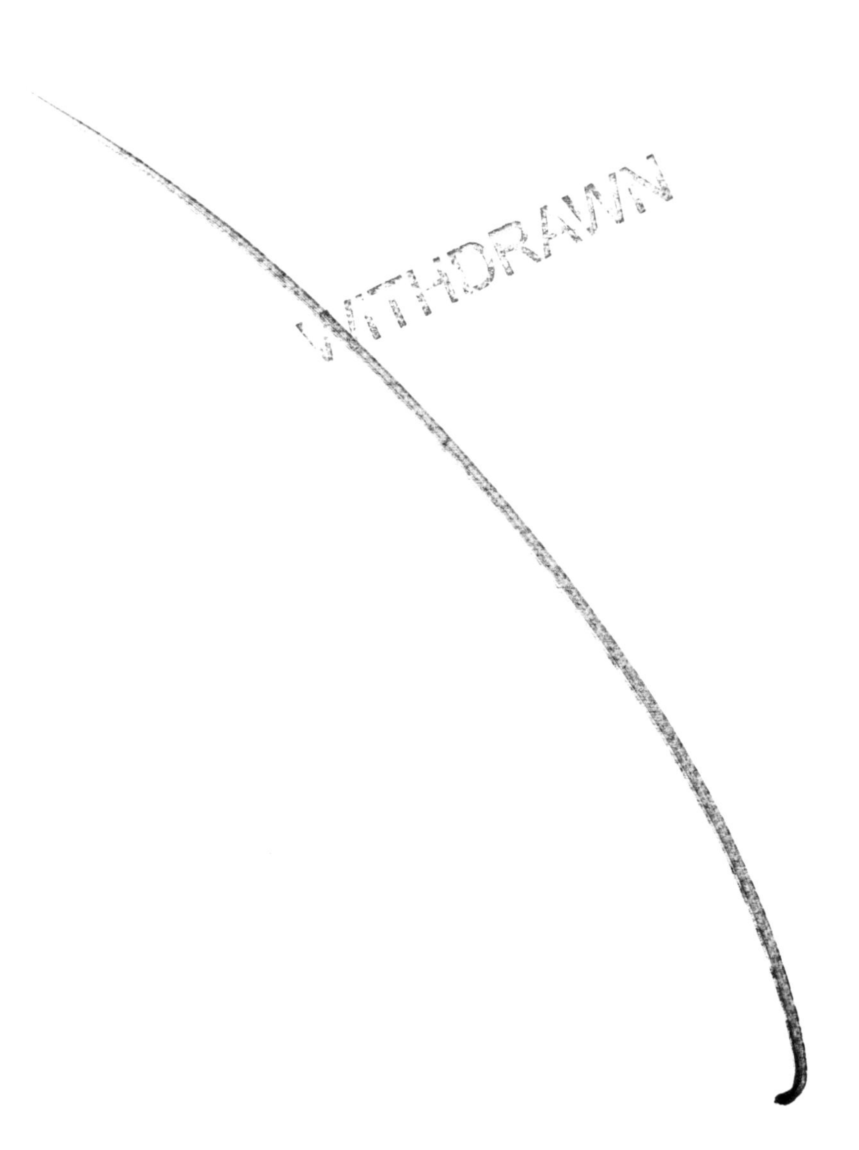

13931626R00076

Made in the USA
Charleston, SC
09 August 2012